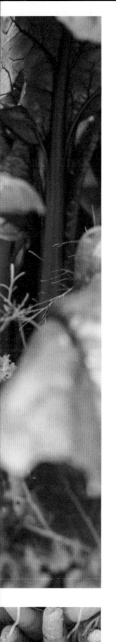
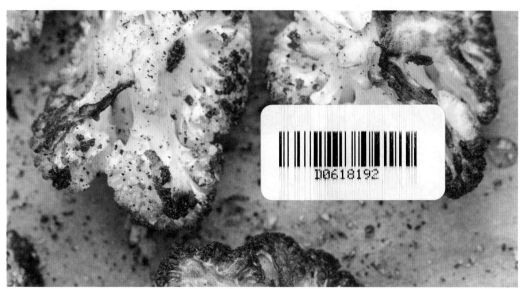
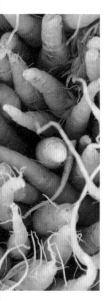
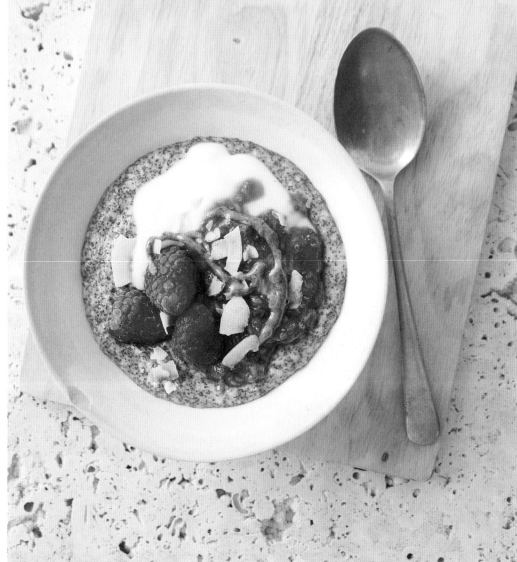

THE
HAPPY
BALANCE

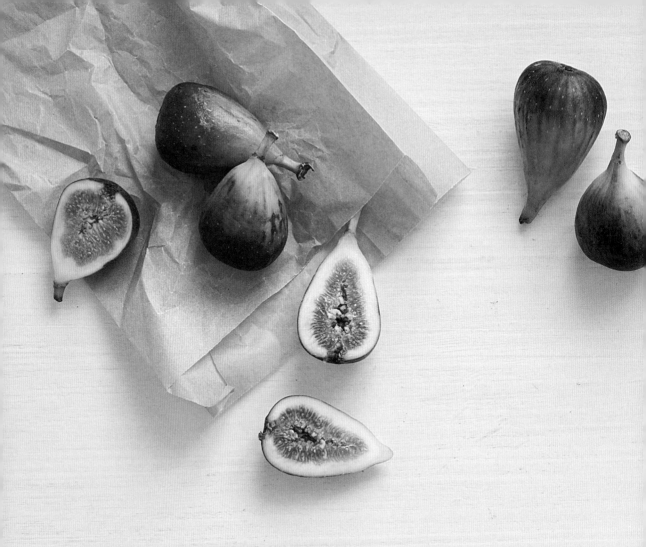

THE HAPPY BALANCE

THE ORIGINAL PLANT-BASED APPROACH FOR HORMONE HEALTH

MEGAN HALLETT
& NICOLE JARDIM

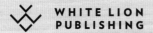
WHITE LION PUBLISHING

CONTENTS

Chapter 4

And Finally

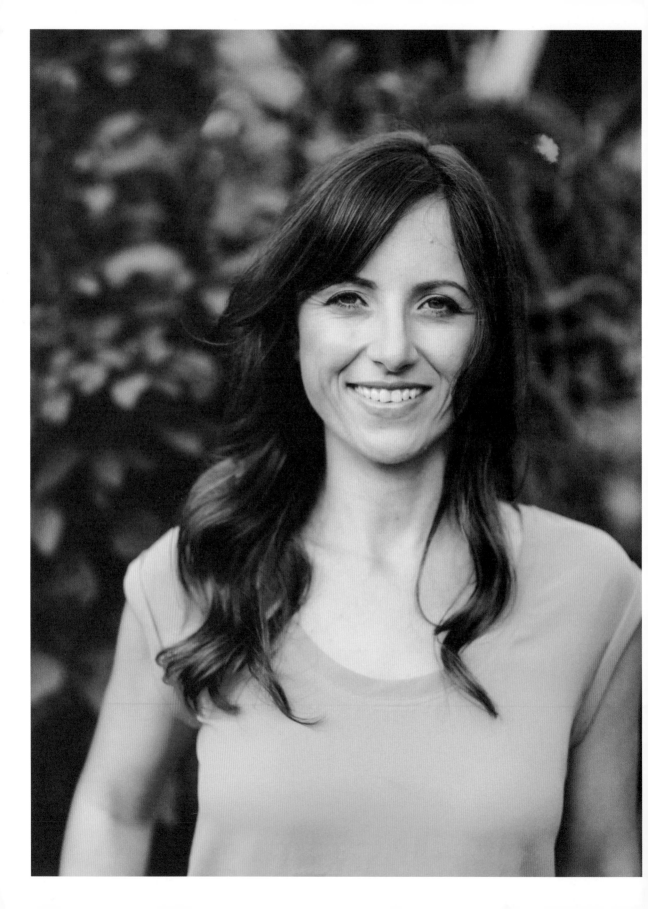

FOREWORD BY NICOLE JARDIM

As a young woman struggling with hormonal imbalance and period problems, I spent years suffering in silence because I thought my experience was just a normal part of life. My mom and most of my friends had suffered terrible teenage periods, which meant I never questioned my own agonisingly painful and heavy cycles.

At 19 my period disappeared for three months, so I made an appointment with my gynaecologist. She immediately prescribed the pill to 'regulate' my cycle. In the first few months of using it I thought I'd found my fix. I spent five years on the pill, and while my periods became lighter and less painful, I started developing a whole host of other serious symptoms including chronic urinary tract and yeast infections, hair loss, joint pain, gut problems and a waning sex drive.

My quest to reclaim my health took me on a multi-year journey that involved countless doctor and specialist visits, often resulting in shrugged shoulders and 'let's wait and see how you feel in six months', endless testing and multiple unnecessary procedures that came back 'normal' or inconclusive.

I was finally referred to an acupuncturist who immediately pointed out that the pill was likely the culprit behind so many of the seemingly unrelated symptoms that I was experiencing. Intuitively, I knew that I was on the right path. Under his care I ditched the pill and overhauled my diet, exercise regimen and lifestyle, which eventually reversed many of the major health problems I'd been experiencing.

The book you are holding in your hands is the life line I was searching for all those years ago. It is exactly what you need if you've been wrestling with the frustrating symptoms of hijacked hormones – period problems, skin issues, weight gain and low energy and sex drive, to name a few.

Megan is uniquely qualified to understand the suffering women experience at the hands of their hormones. She was diagnosed with Polycystic Ovarian Syndrome (PCOS), and like me, had to figure out through trial and error how to naturally fix her own frustrating symptoms.

After experiencing the wellbeing that occurs from having balanced hormones, she felt compelled to train professionally so she could help women in a similar situation to her own. She knew there was a better way than simply taking birth control or medications that only mask the underlying problem.

In *The Happy Balance*, we challenge you to think differently about your hormones and menstrual cycle. Megan takes a multi-faceted approach that includes unbelievably delicious seasonal recipes, addressing sleep, gut and liver health, exercise, low-toxin living and managing our ever-present psychological stress.

We no longer have to accept the hormonal hell that we've been told is just an inevitable part of being a woman. I believe this book is the perfect resource for you as you begin your journey towards achieving hormonal equilibrium.

Nicole Jardim

INTRODUCTION FROM MEGAN HALLETT

From a young age, we're taught to believe that the aches, pains and annoyances of being a woman, are not only completely normal, but expected. Whether you've snapped at your boyfriend for leaving the toilet seat up, or uncontrollably scoffed your way through another giant chocolate bar, we're quick to blame the perplexity we consider our hormones to be.

But what if we took a step back for a moment and had a good think about all of this. It seems that these things have become so accepted as part of what it means to be a woman that we never stop to question this monthly rollercoaster. Yes, sometimes your significant other may just truly wind you up, but how about we stop blaming our hormones for a moment and try to understand these chemical messengers a bit better.

I'm a big believer in taking matters into your own hands and working proactively to balance hormones. In today's world, with the stress and toxins present in everyday life, it is rare you'll find a woman without hormonal issues. Even if you don't know it yet, your body might be giving off help signals that something is not quite right. This could be anything from stubborn weight to acne, anxiety to awful PMS symptoms.

When I was diagnosed with Polycystic Ovarian Syndrome (PCOS), it seemed odd that I was given no information on how to treat this condition naturally, just handed pills to mask the symptoms. Unfortunately, this isn't an uncommon occurrence.

Today, I've managed to soothe my symptoms by nurturing my body through nutrition and lifestyle changes, from stress management to opting for real, whole foods. Through these natural measures, I've cleared up my skin, cured my anxiety, and grown a thick mane after years of my hair thinning. While I am by no means perfect, and my journey is still filled with hiccups, I have become a little hormone obsessed in the process. I've done the research and committed to educating myself on the topic.

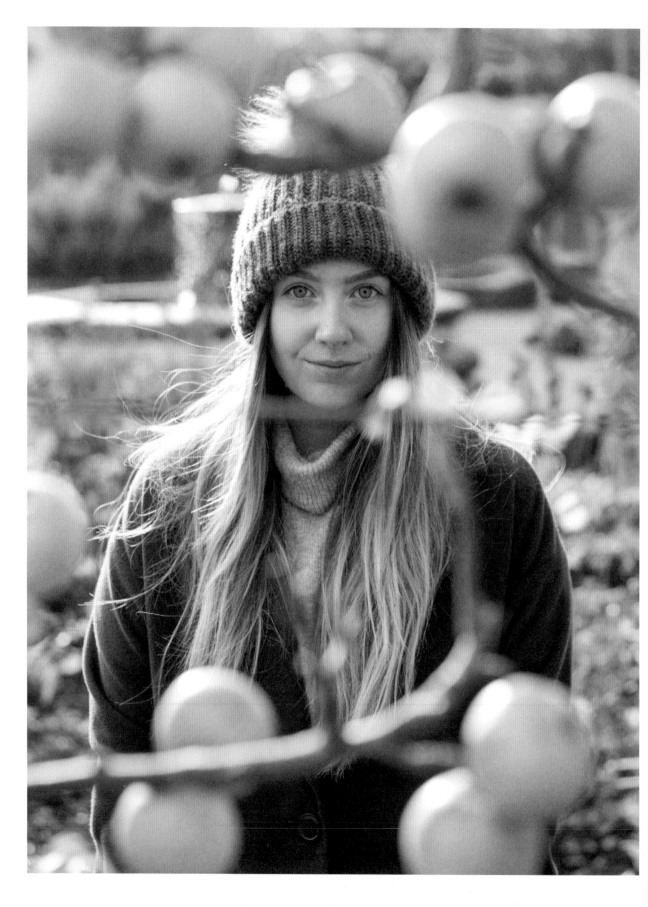

This book is the result of my mission to empower women to reclaim their health and get back in tune with Mother Nature. It is designed to get you thinking of your body as an orchestra, perfectly in sync. You are the front woman, the conductor, keeping everyone, from your adrenals to your detox pathways, playing in time. If the conductor starts to panic, the rest of the orchestra becomes jumbled and messy. But when the conductor is calm and collected, harmony is maintained. A good conductor requires practice, so it may take some time to find what works for you. But you will get there, and your music will be beautiful.

Megan Hallett

HOW TO USE THIS BOOK

The Happy Balance provides all the tools you need to get to know the unique miracle that is your body and hormones. The first step is to understand your body a little better with a crash guide to hormones; the second is to enjoy the delicious plant-based recipes in this book as part of a hormone-healthy lifestyle that will make you glow inside and out. You are welcome!

One of the amazing things about hormones is how much they affect us every day, from puberty through to menopause, and yet how little we know about them. In Chapter One, get to grips with this enigma with a brief guide to what hormones are, how they work and why it matters for our everyday health.

Chapter Two continues the hormone-health 101, introducing the basics of a hormone-healthy lifestyle, from gut health to reducing stress and limiting our exposure to toxins and pollutants. One of the key tenets of a hormone-healthy lifestyle is nutrition, and this chapter delves a little deeper into this, answering the question 'What's food got to do with it?'. Spoiler alert: a lot!

Armed with a new knowledge of hormones and how we can best support our hormone health, you are ready to jump into a hormone-healthy lifestyle and reap the rewards. Start with the delicious plant-based recipes in Chapter Three, all designed to support your body at every stage of its monthly cycle as well as into perimenopause and menopause. You can jump in and choose your favourite recipe, or check out the meal plan (pages 194–197) for a guide to what a hormone-healthy week of meals could look like.

Cycle Syncing

Fluctuating hormone levels mean that our nutritional, exercise and health needs vary at different times of the month. A simple way to optimise our health is to work in tune with these natural rhythms by adapting our diet and exercise regime accordingly. This is called 'cycle syncing'.

Should you want to try cycle syncing, each of the recipes in the book is flagged for the stage it best supports (see key opposite).

For more information on cycle syncing, including how to cycle sync with irregular periods, see pages 39–44.

Recipes for Perimenopause and Menopause

Hormones affect women throughout their lives. The most notable – and notorious – hormonal experience for many is perimenopause and menopause (see page 22). This book will equip you with the information you need not to fear these events, but to recognise them as a new stage in your body's ingenious hormonal journey.

If you are approaching perimenopause and menopause, the recipes in this book provide the best possible nutritional support as well as helping to reduce the often difficult symptoms of this transitional period.

If you are mid-way through perimenopause or menopause, or post-menopausal, you can use the recipes at any time of the month to pack in all the nutrients you need to support your body. Eating in this way is an incredibly powerful tool for health and wellbeing.

Keep it Flexible

The recipes in this book are all plant-based and suitable for a vegan diet. However, a hormone-healthy diet will look different from person to person, and non vegans can easily adapt the recipes in this book. Check out the information on fish, meat and dairy foods on pages 53–55 if you want to include these as part of your hormone-healthy diet.

Key for Cycle Syncing

- Follicular Phase
- Ovulatory Phase
- Luteal Phase
- Menstrual Phase

CHAPTER 1

Hold Up, Hormones?

By Nicole Jardim

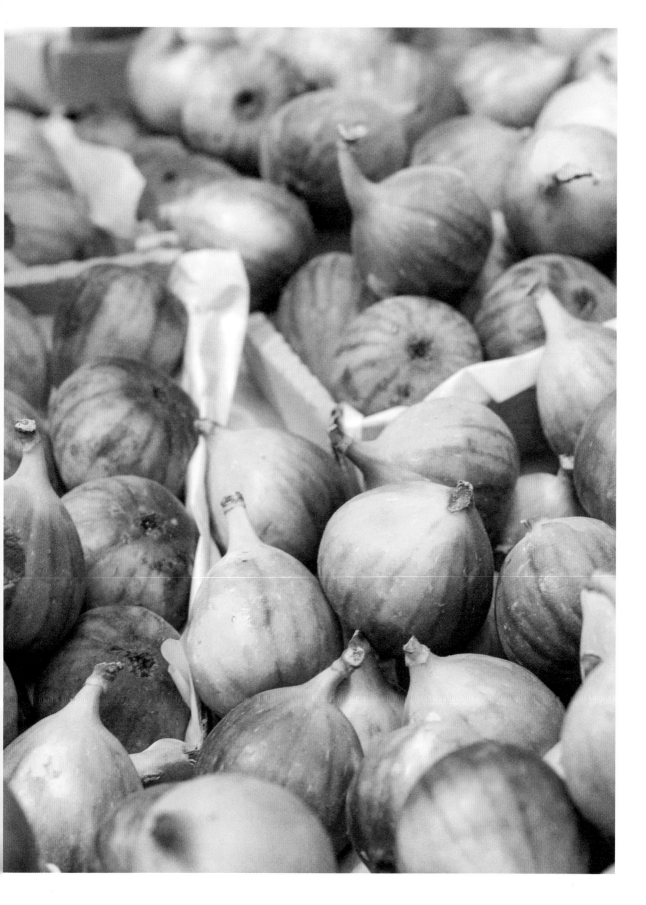

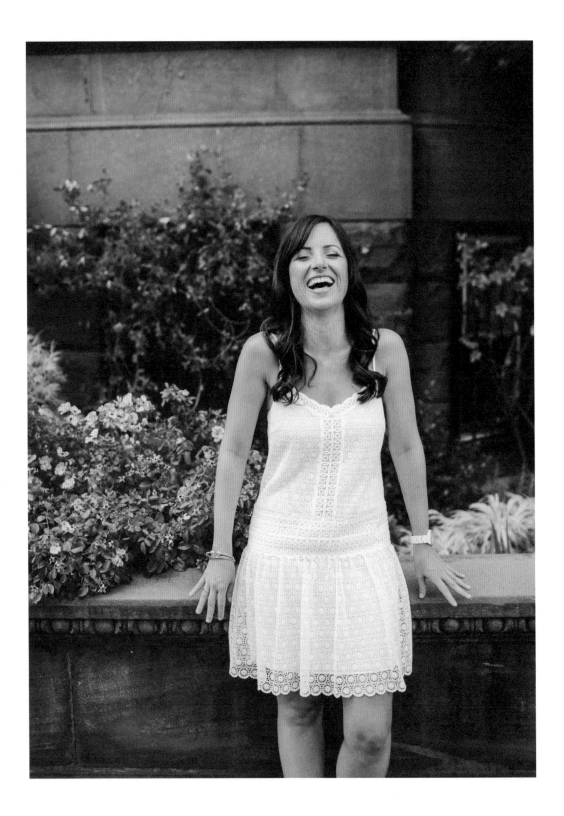

16   The Happy Balance

THE WHAT

Ah, hormones! For most women, the word often evokes images of menopause symptoms, like hot flashes and raging moods. For others, it conjures images of pregnancy and the dreaded premenstrual time of the month.

From birth our hormones are in charge of managing almost all of our bodily functions, including sleep patterns, stress response, emotions, sex drive, appetite and fertility and menstrual cycle function. This is why it's so important for women of every age to have at least a basic awareness and understanding of how our hormones work. Otherwise, we're simply feeling around in the dark, trying to piece together an understanding of what the heck is going on in our bodies and minds.

This confusion about how our bodies function often leads women to feel like they are broken, or that their bodies have somehow failed them. In many cases, they go down a path of unnecessary procedures, medications and hormonal contraception usage to 'treat' symptoms that would be better addressed from the root hormonal cause.

The Endocrine System

So what does an understanding and awareness of our hormones mean? Let's start by looking at the endocrine system. This is a system made up of a group of glands that produce hormones. Hormones are chemical messengers that move throughout the body communicating with other endocrine glands and organs outside this system. The key glands include the hypothalamus and pituitary (both located in the brain), pineal, thyroid, parathyroid, thymus, adrenals, pancreas and ovaries (testes in males). Each of these glands produce hormones that have specific functions in the body.

I like to think of the relationship between the endocrine glands and the hormones as though they are a beautiful symphony: the hypothalamus and pituitary, which are located in the brain, are like the conductors sending 'instruction hormones' to the other endocrine glands throughout the body. The other endocrine glands are the orchestra, receiving these instructions and in response producing their own hormones – the music.

The endocrine glands all have specific hormone receptors that receive the hormone messages. As you can imagine, it's important that they are delivered to the right destination. Think of this as a lock and key situation. Each hormone is like a key for its matching receptor (the lock), binding to the receptor in the same way a key would unlock a door. Once the hormone binds to the receptor, it triggers the desired biological response in the body. This happens thousands of times a day completely unbeknownst to us!

Here are the main glands and hormones we're going to look at:

The pituitary gland produces:

- Follicle stimulating hormone (FSH) and luteinising hormone (LH) – both of which tell the ovaries to start and complete the ovulation cycle each month
- Thyroid stimulating hormone (TSH) – communicates with the thyroid and tells it to produce more or less T3 and T4 (see below)
- Adrenocorticotropic hormone (ACTH) – stimulates the adrenal glands to make their 'stress hormones'.

The pineal gland produces:

- Melatonin – the 'sleepy time' hormone, which dictates our sleep/wake cycle or circadian rhythm.

The thyroid gland produces:

- T4 and T3 – I like to call thyroid hormones the 'go-go-go' hormones because they regulate your energy levels.

The adrenal glands mainly produce:

- The 'stress hormones' cortisol, epinephrine (adrenaline) and norepinephrine
- Dehydroepiandrosterone (DHEA) – helps produce testosterone and oestrogen
- Small amounts of sex hormones.

The pancreas produces:

- Insulin and glucagon – the blood sugar regulating hormones
- Digestive enzymes – to help you break down and digest food.

The ovaries produce:

- Oestrogen, progesterone and testosterone – the key sex hormones.

I'll also touch on other important hormones as they relate to women's health. They include pregnenolone (the 'mother' hormone) and oxytocin (the 'love and bonding' hormone), see page 24.

LIFE STAGES

As you can see, the endocrine system and the myriad of hormones and neurotransmitters produced by it, weave a delicate tapestry of hormonal messages and cellular responses.

Throughout our entire life they are constantly hard at work behind the scenes, which is why I believe managing our hormones at every stage is one of the most important things we women should have on our to-do lists.

Puberty

We don't often realise that imbalances begin long before adulthood. In fact, for many women they show up around the time when puberty starts, so it's critical that young girls are given the education and tools they need to go into this phase of their lives with more empowerment, respect, value and enjoyment for the many gifts of their menstrual cycle.

If you're an adult, you likely remember one – or many! – horror stories about puberty and your first period. One of the first things I'll say about the transition through puberty is that it's important for parents to help girls write a positive period story with rituals, traditions and behaviours that will radically shift how they experience their menstrual cycles into adulthood.

I so often hear from women that their first periods, and that time in their lives in general, were fraught with shame, embarrassment, misunderstanding and low self-esteem. Did you know that young girls' self-esteem plummets at puberty? Not surprising considering our culture of fear and misunderstanding when it comes to how women's bodies function.

So what does a positive period story look like? Opening up the dialogue from an early age – instead of using vague terms like 'private parts', talk about anatomically correct male and female genitalia, and encourage honest discussions about uncomfortable topics like periods and sex if they come up. Celebrate your daughter's first period in a special way so as to validate this as a positive experience for her, and create excitement as she enters adulthood.

Adulthood

Can you imagine entering your late teens and early twenties after having such a positive and affirming experience of puberty and your first period? You'd likely feel way more connection to your body and your menstrual cycle and even potentially experience less hormonal disruption.

It's crucial for adult women to understand that their periods and their fertility are not mutually exclusive entities. Consistent ovulation and a healthy, happy period are signs of optimal fertility, and this is what we should be aiming for every month.

The first step to figuring out your flow is to start tracking your menstrual cycle, ideally using an app on your phone. Track when your period arrives, it's length, and what it looks like. Don't forget to make a note of mood changes, fluctuations in energy levels, sex drive, food cravings, changes in bowel movements and sleep patterns throughout the month. This personal data will help you determine what's normal for your own body.

The next step is to up your nutrition game! We need adequate fat, protein and carbohydrates in order to ovulate each month, which facilitates steroid sex hormone production (oestrogen, progesterone and testosterone to name a few). Some key nutrients that are necessary for healthy hormones and periods include the B-complex vitamins (in particular B6, B9 or folate, and B12), Vitamins A, C, D and E, as well as magnesium, zinc, selenium and iron.

The recipes in this book provide a spectacular array of vitamins and minerals to meet your hormonal health needs. Keep in mind though that B12 is only found in meat, so you must be supplementing with an active form of B12 if you do not eat meat. When I say 'active', I mean a form of B12 that is immediately useable by the body and doesn't have to go through a breakdown process. The active form of B12 is known as methylocobalamin. Additionally, I suggest supplementing with menthylated folate rather than folic acid, I do not recommend folic acid supplementation because many people have a genetic mutation that diminishes their body's ability to break down and utilise folic acid and even folate. Always consult with your doctor before introducing supplements.

Perimenopause and Menopause

One of the biggest myths I'd like to debunk is the idea that menopause is some cliff that we will fall from in the distant future. Real talk ladies – this is just not true.

That's because perimenopause is the transition period between our regular cycling years and the onset of menopause. It's the lead up to our ovaries shuttering their doors for good – that can begin as early as age 35 – where ovulation begins to sputter and women experience sometimes dramatic hormonal changes.

This is why it's so important to take good care of ourselves. Every thing we do, from the food we eat to our exercise regimen over the course of our teens, twenties and thirties, all contribute to what our experience of perimenopause and menopause will be like.

Once our ovaries start winding down egg production, and eventually cease to produce oestradiol and progesterone every month, our lovely adrenal glands take over. They don't produce as much as your ovaries but they are the go-to replacement, and if you've spent the previous three decades in a state of stress overload then your adrenals won't make a great sex hormone surrogate!

Ultimately, most of us are going to head into our perimenopausal years in some state of stress, so don't worry. What matters is you're reading this book right now, which means you'll have the right tools to navigate the perimenopause and menopause.

If you're in your twenties or thirties, following the recipes and advice in this book will set you up for the best possible hormonal journey into perimenopause and menopause. If you have been through, or are currently experiencing, perimenopause or menopause, these recipes can help you to optimize your nutrition for healthy hormone production, supporting overall health and wellbeing.

It is most important for women of any age to focus on regulating their blood sugar and insulin levels, and these recipes are a great place to start. This will go a long way towards managing menopausal symptoms like mood swings, anxiety, fatigue and sleep issues. When our blood sugar levels are wonky from too much sugar and refined flour products, it sends our insulin soaring and then crashing. Insulin is a powerful hormone that impacts your adrenal glands, thyroid and ovaries, thus affecting the hormones produced by these glands.

WHAT IS 'IN BALANCE'?

Nowadays, the term 'hormonal imbalance' is thrown around a lot by people online and in doctor's offices. But what do 'imbalanced hormones' actually mean? These terms are so broad and generalised that most women feel overwhelmed just trying to figure out this first piece of the puzzle.

There are over 50 hormones in the body, but a few main culprits can become imbalanced very easily. The hormones that become imbalanced first are usually cortisol and insulin, the 'stress' and 'blood sugar' hormones produced by the adrenal glands and pancreas respectively. I call these the 'boss lady hormones' because they have a downstream effect on our thyroid, ovarian and sleep hormones. These two hormones effectively regulate how the thyroid hormones, oestrogen, progesterone, testosterone and melatonin all work in the body. If cortisol and insulin become imbalanced or destabilised, then there is a cascade effect on these subordinate hormones.

But what does this mean in terms of symptoms? Here are some of the first signs of cortisol and insulin imbalance to look out for:

- You have trouble falling asleep or you wake up one or more times during the night
- You struggle to get out of bed, even after seven to nine hours of sleep
- You need caffeine just to get going in the morning
- You need more caffeine (or sugar) around 10am and then again at mid-afternoon to keep you going
- You experience mood swings, angry outbursts and energy crashes
- You get 'hangry' more often than you care to admit
- You're putting on weight around your mid-section and you don't know why.

If you experience one or more of these symptoms on a regular basis, you may have imbalanced cortisol or insulin, or both.

You might be thinking 'Really? These are considered symptoms of hormone imbalance?'

I recognise that these symptoms might not seem like issues at all, especially when you consider that downing multiple large coffees a day and burning the midnight oil are pretty common practices in our over-stimulated, high-stress, fast-paced society.

Well, our society is actually part of the problem!

When thinking about cortisol, I want you to visualise it as your body's first line of defence against stress. The moment your brain perceives a threat – whether that is being chased by a lion 100,000 years ago as a hunter/gatherer on the plains of the Serengeti, or in the present day when you're crossing a busy city street and you narrowly avoid being hit by a taxi – your adrenal glands go into overdrive pumping cortisol and epinephrine (adrenaline) directly into your bloodstream.

Both cortisol and epinephrine raise your blood sugar, heart rate and blood pressure, which act like a kind of rocket booster to give you the strength and mental focus to either run or fight.

These stress hormones also prioritise your body's functions, taking off-line non-essentials like your digestive and reproductive systems. I mean, when you're face to face with a lion, getting pregnant or digesting your lunch are not high priorities, right?!

So, in this situation, cortisol just saved your life. Or at least it gave you the best chance to survive. In a split second it turned your body from a complex multi-functioning organism into an efficient focused fighting machine. Pretty cool, huh? So why does this badass hormone get so much bad press?

That brings us back to the present day. The proverbial lion is now chasing our bodies on average about 50 times a day. This comes in the form of overly stressful jobs, relationship problems, chronic illness, malnutrition, financial insecurity, juggling family and work, living in a loud and polluted city...you get where I'm going with this.

Remember what I said about insulin causing problems too? Well, cortisol raises blood sugar, and high blood sugar means higher insulin. Couple that with the fact that far too many of us are eating in a way that destabilises our blood sugar on a daily basis (think excess sugar, refined carbs and even too much protein, which can be converted into sugar) and we find ourselves with chronically high blood sugar, insulin and cortisol.

As you can imagine, when those two boss lady hormones are chronically imbalanced, they are going to wreak hormonal havoc on your DHEA, pregnenolone, oestrogen, progesterone, testosterone, melatonin and thyroid hormones, amongst others.

Here are some of the most common symptoms that you may notice if these other hormones become imbalanced:

- PMS symptoms like breast pain or tenderness, acne, headaches, bloating, irritability and low mood
- Shorter cycles and heavy, painful, more frequent or longer periods; or irregular cycles and lighter, shorter or missing periods
- Lack of desire for sex, and/or painful sex
- Fatigue, brain fog, unexplained hair loss, dry skin and hair, low body temperature (always feeling cold). These symptoms mostly correlate with low thyroid function.
- Diagnosed conditions like Amenorrhea, Adenomyosis, Endometriosis, Graves disease or Hashimoto's Thyroiditis, Infertility, Polycystic Ovarian Syndrome (PCOS), Premenstrual Dysphoric Disorder (PMDD), Premenstrual Syndrome (PMS) and Uterine Fibroids.

That is a whole lot of symptoms from just a few imbalanced hormones! But that's the beauty of hormones. Once you realise that there are just a few key imbalances at the root of a wide variety of symptoms, it makes addressing those symptoms a lot less daunting.

CAUSES OF HORMONAL IMBALANCE

Before we get into solutions, we first have to talk about what causes our hormones to go all haywire in the first place. As I mentioned before, our modern, stressed-out lifestyles can trigger the hormonal avalanche, but what else is messing our hormones about?

Nutrition

First and foremost, we have to look at nutrition, or rather the lack of a nutrient-dense diet, as one of the biggest culprits behind hormonal imbalances. We often forget that everything we consume has either a positive or negative effect on our health. Sugar, refined flour products, excess caffeine and pesticide-laden foods do a real number on our overall health. It's also important to know that you may be eating excellent food but your body might not be breaking it down and absorbing nutrients correctly due to compromised gut health.

Not only that, food sensitivities to gluten, dairy, corn, soy and sugar trigger an inflammatory response that raises your cortisol levels from the inside. So we've got it coming from external and internal sources. Excessive dieting and disordered eating are also extremely taxing on the body, and they must also be addressed as part of a hormone healing plan.

Also don't forget, alcohol raises blood sugar and decreases the liver's detoxification capabilities, which increases oestrogen in the body.

Toxins and Pollutants

Environmental toxins and pollution are massive contributors to our collective hormonal chaos. These include chemicals found in plastic products, makeup and personal care items (body lotion, shampoo and conditioner, hair products and perfume), home cleaning products, pesticides in our foods and toxins in unfiltered drinking water (see page 37).

To give you an idea of what I mean by this, here are a few facts on how toxic chemicals and pollution impact our health:

- Exposure to xenoestrogens (toxic synthetic oestrogens) like BPA (bisphenol A) and phthalates found in plastics, cosmetics and cleaning products contribute to conditions like PCOS, breast cancer and endometriosis (which can cause severe menstrual pain).

- According to the journal *Gynecological Endocrinology*, air pollution significantly impacts fertility in women and is linked to higher rates of miscarriage and lower rates of pregnancy.

Hormonal Birth Control and Other Prescribed Medications

This includes the contraceptive pill, injectable contraceptives and intrauterine devices, as well as certain antibiotics, antidepressants and blood pressure medications. It is extremely important to know that the goal of hormonal birth control is to disrupt your hormones – that is how it works to prevent pregnancy. Without consistent ovulation, a woman's body does not make adequate amounts of oestrogen, progesterone and testosterone and this often leads to irregular periods, or periods that disappear completely, along with mood disorders, acne, hair loss, lowered sex drive, vaginal dryness and more. I recommend women explore natural birth control options like a fertility awareness method (FAM), where women observe and chart their fertility signs throughout their menstrual cycles, or use barrier methods like condoms or diaphragms. Speak to your doctor about which method would work best for you.

With regard to other prescribed medications, I suggest asking your doctor about the potential hormonal side effects before taking them, so that if irregularities crop up, you won't be caught off guard.

Though there are a number of factors that can disrupt our hormonal symphony, there are also many ways to get your hormones back on track. Armed with a little knowledge, you will have a clearer picture of what a hormonal imbalance looks like and how to start to reverse it.

Hormones exist in a hierarchy, so it's important to take a top down approach when it comes to addressing problems that arise from hormonal imbalance. Small shifts in your diet are an excellent place to begin your hormone-healing journey, which is why this book is such a valuable resource. Once you work on your cortisol and insulin, the rest of the subordinate hormones will start to fall in line. That's the beauty of hormones, they are working together to support you.

CHAPTER 2

Balancing Act

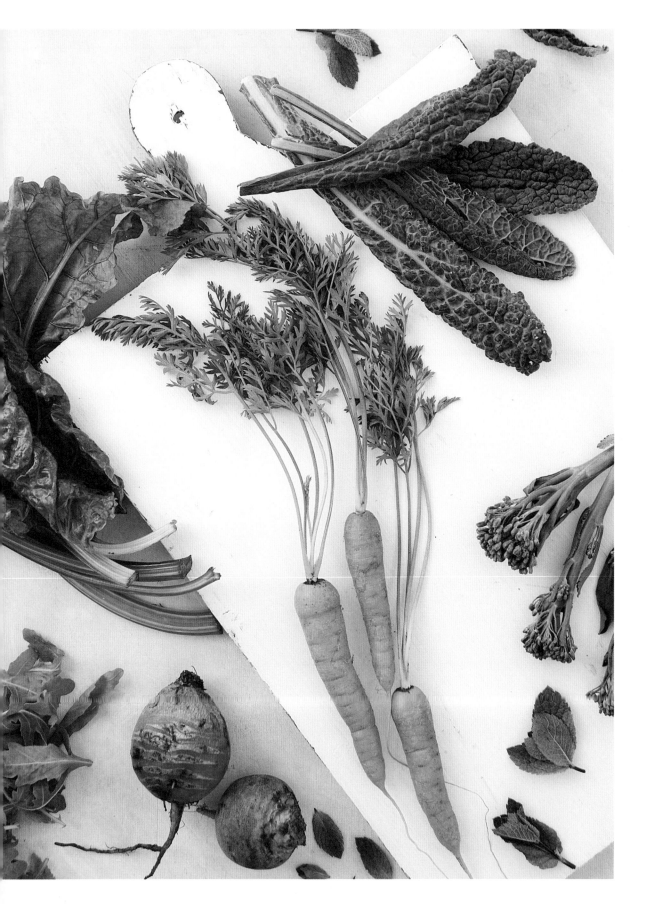

The Healthy Hormone Checklist

By the end of this book, I hope that you'll be a real hormone buff, an expert on what is going on in your body, but for those times when you find yourself a little off balance, refer back to this checklist. The overriding principles of managing your hormone health are very simple: eat real, sleep more, stress less and exercise for your body.

Eat

1. Eat whole, real foods, including lots of healthy fats, and avoid overly proceed foods
2. Hydrate – aim for at least two litres of water (just over eight cups) a day
3. Load up on leafy greens and cruciferous veggies
4. Choose high-quality, organic vegetables, fish and meat, wherever possible
5. Be mindful of caffeine and alcohol intake
6. Limit sugar (of any sort, including unrefined and high-carbohydrate fruits)
7. Limit/avoid refined carbohydrates, such as pasta, bread and pastries
8. Take time over each meal and eat with no distractions
9. Maintain a healthy gut with fermented foods, such as kimchi, sauerkraut and dairy-free coconut yogurt
10. Listen to your body: is gluten or dairy a trigger for you? If so, avoid or limit these in your diet. Everybody is different, so listen to your own unique needs rather than following trends.

Stress and Sleep

1. Organise your diary so that self-care is a priority
2. Meditate every day, even if just for five minutes
3. Get outside – fresh air is essential for our wellbeing
4. Make your bedroom a sanctuary for rest: keep electronic devices outside the bedroom and block all light coming in
5. Turn all screens off one hour before you go to sleep.

Live

1. Prioritise low intensity exercise when getting back into balance
2. Focus on short and sweet HIIT (high-intensity interval training) sessions
3. Invest in natural beauty and cleaning products (see page 37)
4. Avoid buying disposable plastics, and opt for glass where possible. Reusable BPA-free water bottles are a great investment.

THE UNDERDOGS

Your liver and gut are your detox pathways and keeping them in tip-top condition is the key to balanced hormones. The two, combined, are essential cogs in ensuring the body is discarding oestrogen once it's done its job. If not appropriately dealt with, this hormone can re-circulate and lead to oestrogen dominance, which causes bloating, stubborn weight around the middle and mood swings, to name a few.

Gut Health

A healthy gut, more often than not, means a healthy body. The gut underpins everything, from the production of serotonin to happy hormones. Ensuring that you are having regular and healthy bowel movements can be overlooked but is absolutely essential to our digestive health.

One simple way to improve gut health is to take more time over our meals. The urgency of everyday life means we rarely do this. Turn the television off while you are eating and put your phone away – this is a simple concept that makes a real difference.

There are also some great gut-friendly foods that can help. Establish a healthy environment in your gut with prebiotic rich foods, such as asparagus, artichokes and onions. Then maintain that environment with fermented foods that feed the good bacteria, such as sauerkraut, kimchi and kombucha.

Ayurvedic Principles

If you are at your wits end with your digestion, look to Ayurveda, an ancient Eastern philosophy that puts digestion and balance at the heart of everything. Cook with wonderfully warming spices to keep your digestive system ablaze, avoid drinking lots of water with meals and, where possible, drink it warm instead.

Ayurveda teaches us to follow the seasons: slurping frozen smoothies in the middle of winter may not be what your body needs at that point in time, so opt for comforting breakfast bowls instead.

Liver Health

All the fun things – alcohol, caffeine and sugar – can be described as 'liver loaders', as they distract the liver from doing its job. Of course, we're all here to live our best lives, and sometimes that consists of sipping proseccos at sunset with your friends. However, it is something to be conscious of if you are struggling with symptoms of imbalance. That might mean savouring just the one glass, rather than half a bottle – or opting for alcohol-free alternatives that can feel just as indulgent.

Incorporating overflowing handfuls of dark leafy greens into every meal can help support your liver. As can eating a range of whole, real foods, investing in a vitamin B supplement (see page 52) and sipping on herbal teas such as dandelion, milk thistle and burdock. And lastly, drink water: two litres a day at the very least; filtered is always best.

LIVING WELL

Hormone health is about more than nutrition and digestion. In order to keep our hormones in check – including the stress hormone, cortisol – we need to make sure our lifestyle is hormone-healthy, too. This includes practicing regular self-care, prioritising good sleep, exercising regularly and avoiding toxins where possible.

Dealing with Stress

We live in a world where busy is the new norm, and we take pride in telling others just how exhausted we are. Yet in the midst of this, self-care is absolutely essential in maintaining optimal health. Self-care isn't just having a bath when life gets too much, it's organising your life so it doesn't get to that point. How can you expect to give something your all, when you haven't got it all to begin with?

Set aside time every day to switch off from other cares and concerns. Delete Instagram for a couple of days and listen to podcasts instead. Indulge in an evening of Friends re-runs and have a Golden Coconut Milk (see page 138). Build a huge stack of cookbooks beside your bed and don't get up you've gone through them all. Everyone is different, so whatever soothes your soul and puts you into a state of complete and utter calm: do it.

In reality, stressful things do happen, and sometimes there is nothing you can do about it. You can't control the external stressors, but you can control how you respond to them. When it comes to adjusting your response to things, be strict on yourself. Set a firm 'no discussing work at the dinner table' rule, tackle challenges with a positive attitude and practice meditation regularly, so that mindfulness becomes integrated into your everyday life.

Sleep

Sleep is a fundamental part of health, and there are studies upon studies showing that the quality of your sleep is just as, if not more, important than the length of your sleep. You can be in bed for hours on end, but unless you are in that lovely deep state of REM sleep (that dreamy state where your body is in full recovery mode), your cortisol isn't given enough of a chance to reach a healthy level. Your head should hit the pillow feeling calm and in need of a good re-charge and waking up should have you feeling fresh and ready to take on the day. However, the opposite of this is often more common an occurrence.

Sleep hygiene is essential for maintaining optimal hormone balance and includes creating a relaxing and restful bedroom environment, as well as a nourishing night-time routine. Long story short, your circadian rhythm (a twenty-four-hour cycle that regulates various bodily functions) comes down to the way sunlight effects your rising and rest. It's how the external influences your internal sense of structure and schedule. Commit to all screens off at least one hour before bedtime and make this time the relaxing end to your day. The blue light from our devices is a major endocrine disruptor and lowers melatonin levels in the body, which we need to drift off into a restful slumber.

If you're getting your cycle back on track, then a healthy production of melatonin, the sleep hormone, is vital for both your circadian rhythm and healthy balance of oestrogen and progesterone.

Here are some simple yet effective ways to achieve better quality sleep:

1. Switch off all screens at least one hour before bedtime and make the bedroom a device-free environment
2. Keep a regular sleep/wake rhythm, even on weekends
3. If you are still having trouble drifting off, accept a helping hand from sleepy herbs and teas, such as good old camomile, valerian, ashwagandha or CBD oil, or try the Soothing Lavender Bedtime Milk on page 143
4. Scatter magnesium flakes into a warm bath before bedtime
5. Diffuse essential oils by the side of your bed (such as lavender, ylang-ylang and neroli), invest in a pillow spray and smother your body in lavender-infused butter.

Move It

Endophins are the wonderful mood-boosting hormones released when we exercise, so find a way of moving that feels good for you at that moment in time.

Yoga and Pilates are two fabulous low-intensity classes you can take if you are trying to get your hormones back on track and keep overworked adrenals happy. Walking and swimming are also a great way to combine exercise and daily meditation: bonus points if you can get outside and do them in nature.

For the times in your cycle where you are bursting with energy, head out on a run, hit the gym or attend a fun class. But always examine how your body is feeling and adjust your workouts accordingly.

Live Clean: Toxins in Beauty Products

Green beauty is not only one of the best things we can do for
our planet, it's also incredibly important for our health. We're
hyper aware of what we put into our bodies, but what about
what we put on to them? As skin is transdermal (meaning it is
permeable), we need to ensure we're mindful about ingredients
that can shake up our endocrine system in the same way that
stress and food can. This includes anything from deodorant
to what you're cleaning your kitchen floor with. Here are a few
common culprits to be mindful of:

Deodorant – the skin under your arms is extremely thin
and highly absorbent, and there are a number of harmful
substances in your standard deodorants, including aluminum.
Look out for natural brands like Salt of the Earth and Schmidts.

Sanitary products – your vagina is lined with highly porous
mucous membrane, so go organic and avoid scented products.

Foundation, body lotion and sunscreen – if it's going
directly onto your skin, be extra mindful of the ingredients that
are in it.

Facial cleansers and moisturisers – a good skincare brand
will be transparent about their ingredients and are free from
endrocrine disruptors including parabens, phthalates,
fragrances and silicones. Sukin is a fabulous brand, as is
Herbivore and my personal favourite, Drunk Elephant.

Mascara and eyeliner – the skin around your eye is another
highly absorbent area, so pay attention to the products you are
applying here and prioritise natural, organic ingredients.

Toothpaste and mouthwash – there are some truly great
products out there to keep you minty fresh, such as Kingfisher,
Georganics and Green People, so you don't have to worry about
this one.

Shampoo, conditioner and styling products – opt for coconut or jojoba oil for a wonderfully moisturising natural hair mask. Products can easily be absorbed through your scalp, so, as with the rest of your beauty regime, avoid endocrine-disrupting ingredients including phthalates and parabens. The latter is known to have oestrogen-mimicking properties, something we want to avoid putting onto and into our bodies.

Air fresheners – plug-in air fresheners can be extremely hormone disruptive and can enter the body in a multitude of different ways. Diffuse some essential oils instead.

Household cleaning products – products such as washing up liquid, surface cleaner and floor cleaner can all contain harsh chemicals so look out for natural and organic brands that are softer on both you and the environment.

IN SYNC

At first, the concept of cycle syncing might sound a little ludicrous, however, when you think about it, it really does make sense. After all, you are essentially a completely different person during each phase of your cycle, so why would you eat, move and live the same way throughout? Adapting what you're putting into your body, and how you're utilising it, allows you to be the very best version of yourself at any given time during your cycle.

So, why should you be cycle syncing and who is it particularly helpful for? Zoning in on each specific phase of your cycle gives you a real awareness of your body and is helpful in restoring hormonal balance and establishing a healthy cycle post birth control, as well as tackling any painful PMS. It also provides invaluable knowledge when prepping your body for conception, be it in the near or distant future, and even to restore a slight sense of structure during the perimenopause phrase.

Throughout the book, recipes are flagged for which cycle phase they will be particularly nourishing for. However, try not to get too bogged down on being perfect with this. Focus more on nourishing and moving your body in a way that makes you feel happy.

On the following pages, you'll find a quick breakdown of each phase of the cycle and what it means for your body.

Follicular Phase

Energy levels start to peak post menstruation, as do testosterone and oestrogen levels, so use this time to get stuff done. Within your body, follicles in your ovaries that house your eggs will start to blossom once again, one of which will take the lead and release an egg at ovulation. This egg has the potential to be fertilised if it comes into contact with sperm once it has been released by the follicle. As the name suggests, this phase is all about nourishing those follicles that are vital for healthy ovulation.

Eat: Pack in those follicle nourishing fats, folate and vitamin E to help build and maintain a healthy lining in your uterus. Think an avocado a day and lots of homemade nut butter – in smoothies or spooned straight from the jar. Opt for foods that help promote oestrogen metabolism, such as broccoli, sprouts and cabbage.

Follicular meals to try:
Roasted Fennel, Rocket and Wild Rice Salad (see page 94)
No Nonsense Plant-based Butters (see page 180)
Green Coriander Cream Dressing (see page 186)

Move: Use this surge of energy to head to that dance cardio class you've been eyeing all month, and get lifting those heavy weights. The high oestrogen and testosterone circulating throughout your body are great for building muscle mass.

Ovulatory Phase

It's not uncommon to feel a little bloated and puffy during the ovulatory phase, and during the releasing of the egg, you might feel a slight lower abdominal cramp known as mittelschmerz, or pain in the middle. At the same time, you're likely to be feeling a little more sociable during this time as oestrogen levels peak, due to your body naturally wanting to partner up and reproduce.

Eat: Fermented and fibre-rich foods support healthy digestion and flush away excess oestrogen. Support your liver by loading up on dark leafy greens and sipping on detoxifying herbal teas. Be extra mindful about drinking at least two litres of filtered water a day, and perhaps lay off the alcohol, caffeine and sugar.

Ovulatory meals to try:
Liver-Supporting Green Juice (see page 65)
Overnight Teff Breakfast Bowl (see page 74)
Zesty Chargrilled Broccoli (see page 135)

Move: Combine long hikes with a good natter with your girl friends. Fill your diary with group classes such as Pilates or a motivational spin class, a perfect way to merge that urge to be extra social with keeping fit.

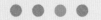

Luteal Phase

If your egg hasn't been fertilised, then your body is in menstruation preparation mode once again, and as testosterone and oestrogen levels drop, progesterone levels rise. Many women experience mood swings during this phase, but you can combat that by keeping your blood sugar stable.

Eat: Now's the time for comfort food and dishes that will continue to support your liver: think large stews full of lentils and leafy greens. If you're craving chocolate, enjoy until your heart's content – cacao is rich in magnesium, fabulous for combating fatigue, as are pumpkin seeds and spinach. Certain foods, including fermented foods, help the natural production of serotonin, which will help ease sudden shifts in mood, so pile your plate high with quinoa, buckwheat and sauerkraut.

Luteal meals to try:
Delicata Squash and Black Rice Salad (see page 96)
Chocolate and Cardamom Nourish Balls (see page 147)
Nut-free Salted Chocolate Tart (see page 158)

Move: Fatigue is your body crying out for you to take it easy, so enjoy yoga, swimming and find solace in long walks accompanied by happy-music playlists and hilarious podcasts.

Menstrual Phase

And finally, the menstrual phase, also known as 'that time of the month'. Progesterone levels drop and this triggers the release of the uterine lining. Enjoy this time to kick back and let your body do its thing, then enjoy the surge of energy as you swing back around into your follicular stage.

Eat: Stock up on anti-inflammatory staples, incorporating them into your meals by sipping on golden milk, chai lattes and loading curries with wonderfully warming spices. Nourish yourself with stews, soups and dahl. Reach for foods rich in iron – adding dried kombu or wakame into simmering saucepans of grains is a great way to do this.

Menstrual meals to try:
Healing Shiitake Mushroom Miso Soup (see page 101)
Beetroot and Portobello Mushroom Stew (see page 116)
Golden Coconut Milk (see page 138)

Move: Do restorative yoga, go for walks in nature and, towards the end of your period when you start feeling like your usual self again, a light jog will help with any cramping you might be experiencing. It's okay to avoid hectic gyms and overcrowded classes at this time, as your typically social self may not be feeling up to it, so enjoy time alone if you so wish.

Irregular cycle?

If you have been experiencing an irregular cycle, you can still cycle sync by following the lunar calendar below. Whether you've recently transitioned off birth control, or you suffer from a condition such as PCOS, instead of merely guessing whereabouts in your cycle you are, let the moon determine. For some women, this can be really useful for getting back in sync.

Waxing crescent to waxing quarter – Follicular
Full moon – Ovulation
Waning quarter to waning crescent – Luteal
New moon/no moon – Menstruation

If you are using the moon phases as a guide, ensure you're aware of each phase through the use of a lunar calendar and giving the moon a quick glance every night. Honour your natural circadian rhythm by being mindful of screen use around bedtime, as the light is endocrine disruptive and can affect re-establishing a natural cycle.

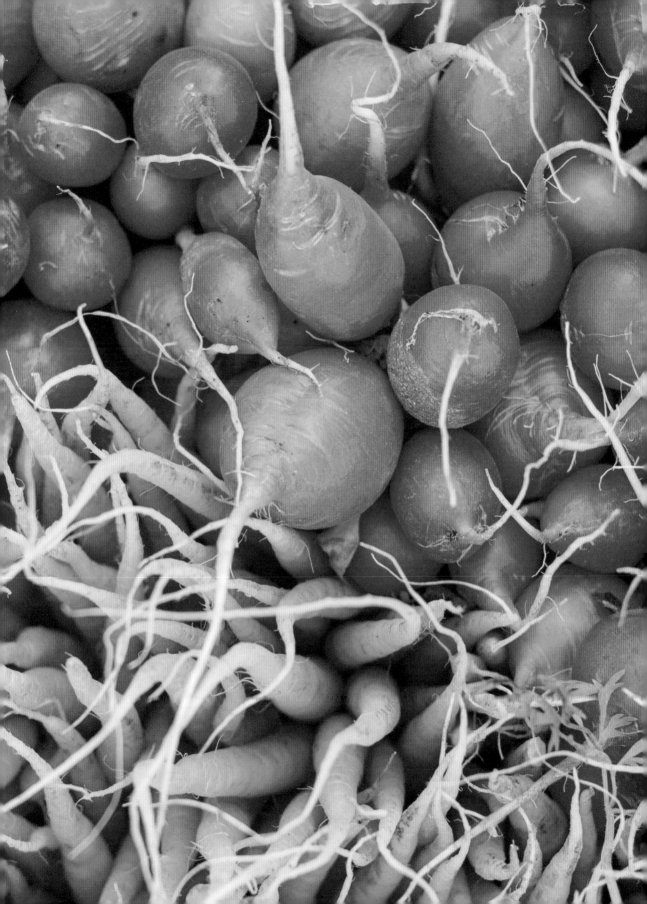

EVERYDAY SUPER FOODS

It feels strange calling any particular food 'super', as to be honest, anything in the right moment could be considered so. From a pint of chocolate ice cream after a nasty break up to a hearty sweet potato stew on a cold evening – both can be considered super if they set your soul alight at that very moment. However, this is a hormone-balancing book, so let's chat about some of the amazing ingredients that can give you a helping hand. Super foods don't have to be hard-to-come-by dusts and tinctures, sometimes a super food is a humble strawberry or a handful of greens.

Dark Leafy Greens
Liver-supporting leafy greens include spinach, kale, cavolo nero, chard and mustard greens – all great sources of folic acid, magnesium and calcium. Cram them into every meal, from a couple of frozen spinach cubes in a morning smoothie to generous handfuls in stews.

Cruciferous Vegetables
Broccoli, cauliflower and cabbage are a few of the most common cruciferous vegetables and are all super easy to incorporate into meals. Grill or lightly steam Tenderstem broccoli for a simple side dish and scoff fermented sauerkraut to reap cabbage's oestrogen-metabolising benefits.

Avocado
Avocados are rich in monounsaturated fat and folate, both essential for your hormones. Smashed over warm sourdough or tossed into salads are both delicious ways to enjoy this creamy powerhouse. Try cooking with avocado oil, as it has a high smoke point, meaning you maintain all the lovely health benefits.

Dairy-free Coconut Yogurt, Butter and Milk
Thick and creamy coconut yogurt dolloped over berries is guaranteed to fill even the emptiest of bellies and stabilise blood sugar. Coconut

products taste so indulgent, from butter to milk, and are great plant-based alternatives to everyday staples.

Herbal Tea

Herbal teas can be a great tool to use alongside a healthy diet and useful in supporting your detox pathways (particularly dandelion and milk thistle). Raspberry leaf can help to promote a healthy cycle and spearmint has been known for its anti-androgen properties, which is helpful for women with PCOS.

Quinoa and Gluten-free Grains

As plants go, quinoa is high in protein and contains a good amount of fibre, great for maintaining healthy digestion. From black rice, teff, millet, amaranth and buckwheat, to humble oats, cook your hearty whole grains into warming breakfast bowls or layer underneath fiery veggie curries. A cupboard well stocked with grains means you'll always have something to eat.

Sweet Potatoes

It's important to cram a range of complex carbohydrates into each day, and sweet potatoes make doing so a breeze. They're fibre rich, high in vitamin E (hello healthy skin) and vitamin C, essential for healthy progesterone levels.

Nuts, Nut Butters and Seeds

Nuts and seeds are a great way to pack in those healthy fats, whether you're nibbling on-the-go or adding generous spoonfuls of almond butter to smoothies. Pumpkin and sesame seeds are rich in magnesium too, which is essential for supporting a healthy cycle and battling fatigue.

Berries

Strawberries, blueberries and raspberries are all fabulous nutritious gems as they are antioxidant packed and low in sugar, meaning they won't spike your blood glucose levels the way that bananas and other high-carbohydrate fruits such as mangos can.

Sea Veg

Dried seaweed is a great, yet largely overlooked cupboard staple. Reach for dulse, kombu, kelp or wakame during your menstrual phase for an iron boost.

A high-quality plant-based protein powder, such as hemp, pea or brown rice, can be a great addition to your diet, and easily blended into smoothies or mixed into porridge. Ensure the list of ingredients is short and free from any added sugar or stabilisers.

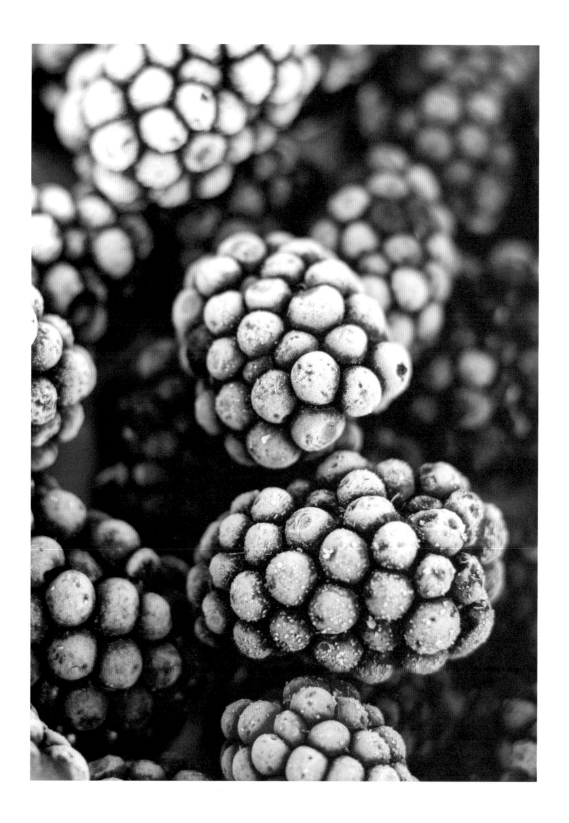

POSSIBLE AGGRAVATORS

When it comes to food, we should celebrate ingredients instead of fear mongering. However, when things get rough and your hormones feel chaotic, taking things back to basics could be just what your body needs. Learn what works for you, but the following foods are those that typically aggravate hormones the most.

Sugar

Includes: fruit juice, artificial sweeteners, refined sugar and, in some cases, too many unrefined sources, such as certain fruits.

As fun as sugar may be, cutting your intake down can have incredible effects on your hormones, as you'll avoid drastic blood sugar spikes that have a knock-on affect on the rest of your hormones.

How to get around this: cook with dates instead – you'll be packing in the fibre alongside the sweetness.

Fake Food

Includes: meal replacement shakes and bars and packaged foods with lengthy ingredient lists.

When you're short on time, a ready meal can seem heaven sent. In order to restore harmony among your hormones, if you are choosing a ready meal, make sure that you opt for real, whole ingredients, and ensure that you check and understand the full ingredient list for the food you're eating.

How to get around this: build meals using foods from the ground rather than from a box, experiment in the kitchen and discover recipes you love. Look for recipes that you can prep ahead or make in bulk then freeze for quick weekday options.

High GI Foods

Includes: bread, pasta and pastries.

White flour can have a similar effect on our bodies as sugar. That being said, please don't skimp on the pasta if you find yourself on a once-in-a-lifetime trip to Italy. Enjoy the simplicity of the dishes made from fresh, local ingredients.

How to get around this: walk into a health-food store and find shelves full of different types of pastas staring back at you, from black bean fettuccine to chickpea fusilli.

Dairy

Includes: milk, yogurt, cheese.

Dairy can be a major culprit in throwing you off-balance if you have underlying issues to begin with. This is due to both synthetic and natural hormones in a lot of the milk on our shelves today.

How to get around this: head to pages 178–179 for my favourite plant-based milk recipes.

Caffeine and Alcohol

Of course, we're all entitled to a drink here and there, and sometimes deadlines and late nights send you crawling towards the closest coffee shop. Just be conscious of the effect that stimulants like these have on your body when trying to restore balance, as they do trigger blood sugar spikes and also put a lot of pressure on your liver.

How to get around this: two words: mocktails and matcha.

IN ADDITION

Women often ask me if supplements are a necessary part of daily life. The answer to that is yes, because our soils are depleted due to intensive farming and so our food is lacking in key nutrients. We're also not eating as varied a diet as our ancestors did, and many of us are over-stressed and sleep-deprived. Not a great combination!

For these reasons, I highly recommend women include these supplements for optimal hormonal health:

Magnesium

This mineral plays a vital role in supporting the nervous system and helps prevent anxiety, nervousness, restlessness and irritability. Sufficient magnesium improves PMS symptoms like migraines and bloating in particular. Magnesium also improves insulin sensitivity, meaning that your body is better able to use insulin to regulate your blood sugar. This is especially helpful for women who are predisposed to blood sugar irregularities and women with PCOS.

B Complex

The B Complex of vitamins, which includes B1, B2, B3, B5, B6, B9 and B12 are amazing for a variety of hormonal imbalances and period-related problems. These include abnormal bleeding or spotting, heavy periods, fibrocystic breasts, endometriosis and menstrual cramps (B1 and B3 in particular). And B1, B2 and B6 can significantly lower your chance of having PMS. Additionally, B6 helps detox oestrogen from the body and lower prolactin (high levels can inhibit ovulation).

Omega-3 Fish Oil or Cod Liver Oil

If you are vegan or vegetarian, you can include an algae-based Omega-3 supplement in your diet. Omega-3 fatty acids DHA and EPA are anti-inflammatory rockstars. They can improve pain associated with menstrual cramps, migraines, endometriosis and fibromyalgia. Omega-3's also help improve PMS symptoms.

A Note from Nicole on Dairy

I've found cow's milk dairy products to be problematic for most women, often contributing to period pain and endometriosis, heavy periods, PMS and PMDD, and acne or other skin conditions. This is because cow's milk contains a protein known as A1 casein, which can trigger inflammation in the body. So, if you had childhood issues, such as lots of colds or ear infections, then it was likely caused by a dairy intolerance or allergy. As adults, it can show up as stomach aches, IBS symptoms like chronic constipation or diarrhea, a stuffy or runny nose, or feeling phlegmy after you eat it. If you're in menopause, it's worthwhile looking out for these symptoms or trying to think back to when you were younger and figuring out whether you had those period or childhood problems. Dairy products from goat or sheep's milk are usually okay because they contain A2 casein, which does not have the same inflammatory effect on the body. Also, butter does not contain much A1 casein, so you may find you have no issues with it.

If you experience any of these symptoms, I recommend that you remove all types of dairy for 28 days and see if your cycle-related symptoms improve. Not everyone is sensitive to A1 dairy, but it's important to learn if you are, as part of your hormone-balancing regimen. Women can often reintroduce goat or sheep's milk dairy products without a problem.

A Note from Nicole on Protein

Protein is the main structural building block of our hormones, and without it our endocrine system would cease to function. Additionally, women need a specific set of nutrients in order to ovulate consistently, including adequate complete protein (protein sources containing all 8 amino acids), zinc, selenium, iron, iodine, omega 3 fatty acids, vitamin B12 and vitamin A (the preformed type called retinol, which is found primarily in liver, kidney and egg yolks, is most easily absorbed and utilised by the body). Plant sources contain carotenoids which need to be converted into a useable form of vitamin A. Some plant sources include sweet potatoes, butternut squash, carrots, mangos, pumpkins, kale, spinach and collard greens. These nutrients collectively contribute to overall health and, ultimately, consistent ovulation.

Meat and fish provide good sources of animal protein; always choose organic, farm-raised and grass-fed meat, free-range eggs and wild-caught fish, where possible. Plant-based sources of protein include nuts, seeds and legumes such as beans and lentils , which also contain some B vitamins, vitamin E, magnesium, selenium, zinc and a little iron.

I want you to think of protein as a side, versus the main part of your meals. It really should only take up a quarter of your plate, with the rest of your meal consisting of vegetables and healthy fats.

FLEXIBLE OPTIONS

The recipes in this book are all plant-based, reflecting the way I love to eat. However, that doesn't mean you have to be strict when following each recipe. Feel free to customise them depending on your flexitarian, pescatarian or meat-eater needs. Perhaps you want to add salmon alongside one of the hearty salads, or top your avo toast with a poached egg. As Nicole says: vibrant veggies and healthy fats should always make up the majority of your meal with protein accounting for one quarter of plate. For now, here's a cheat sheet on hormone-healthy fish sources, with cooking instructions based on one to two portions:

Good Fish Sources

Salmon A great source of Omega-3 fatty acids, salmon is known for its brain boosting properties and couldn't be easier to cook. Simply bake for 15 minutes at 180°C/350°F/gas mark 4. Alternatively you can steam, in foil over gently simmering water for just under 10 minutes alongside the rest of your vegetables. Always opt for wild caught.

Cod This packs a real punch on the protein scale and has a subtle flavour makes it a fail-safe accompaniment for most meals. It's rich in vitamin B12 and can be quickly pan-fried for 3–4 minutes on each side over a medium heat in avocado oil; or bake in a baking parcel (see below) for 10 minutes at 180°C/350°F/gas mark 4.

Mackerel This oily fish is another Omega-3 hero. Mackerel can be a welcome addition to your diet for its B-vitamins alone, as well as its healthy skin benefits. Season the fillets and fry in a pan with a dash of avocado oil for no more than 5 minutes on a medium heat.

Short on time? Place your fish of choice into a baking parchment parcel along with any herbs, lemon or vegetables, and season with salt and pepper. Serve up alongside the Roasted Fennel, Rocket and Wild Rice Salad (page 94), or the easy Grilled Courgette, Asparagus and Rocket Salad (page 95).

HAPPINESS

While writing this book I've come to the realisation that happiness is everything. You can eat hormone-balancing superfoods to your heart's content, but if doing so causes you immense stress, then forget those super benefits. Your mind shouldn't become a war zone when thinking about nutrition, and choosing to grab an ice cream on the first sweltering day of summer shouldn't come at the cost of days of guilt. Overthinking your food choices can, and will be, worse for your body than that cupcake ever will be. So calm down, you're doing just fine.

Enjoy your food because it feeds every cell in your body the love and nutrients they deserve. Make healthy choices because you want to feel amazing, not just look amazing and so that you can be the powerful, unstoppable force of nature you already know you are. This book is designed to guide you through the ups and downs of being a woman and give you the nutrition and lifestyle advice you need to shine, inside and out. Part of this involves listening to your body's cues: we're all different and learning what works for you is incredibly empowering.

And lastly, surround yourself with those who will say you absolutely *can* when you think you *can't*, who pick you up when you're feeling down, and truly get what you're going through during the times when womanhood feels like one giant calamity. Your support network can have a major effect on your overall health, so choose wisely and once you've found them, never let them go.

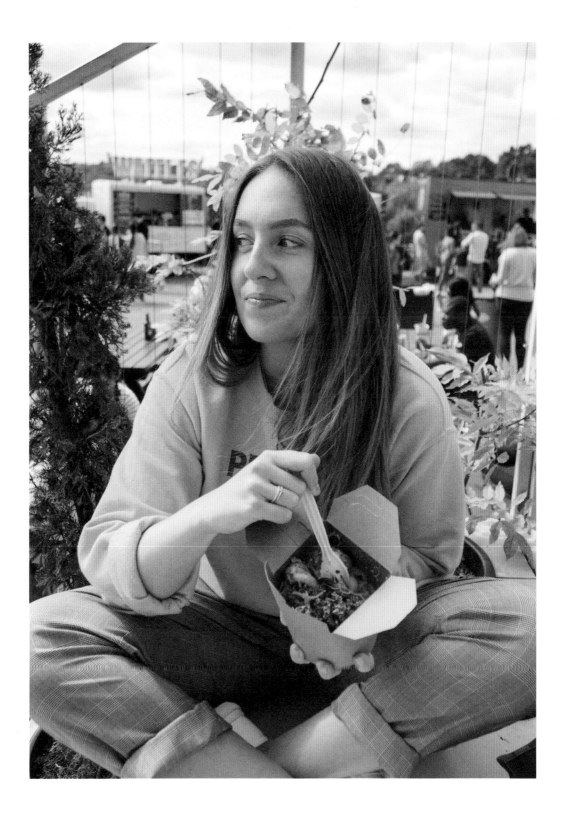

CHAPTER 3

Right, Now I'm Hungry

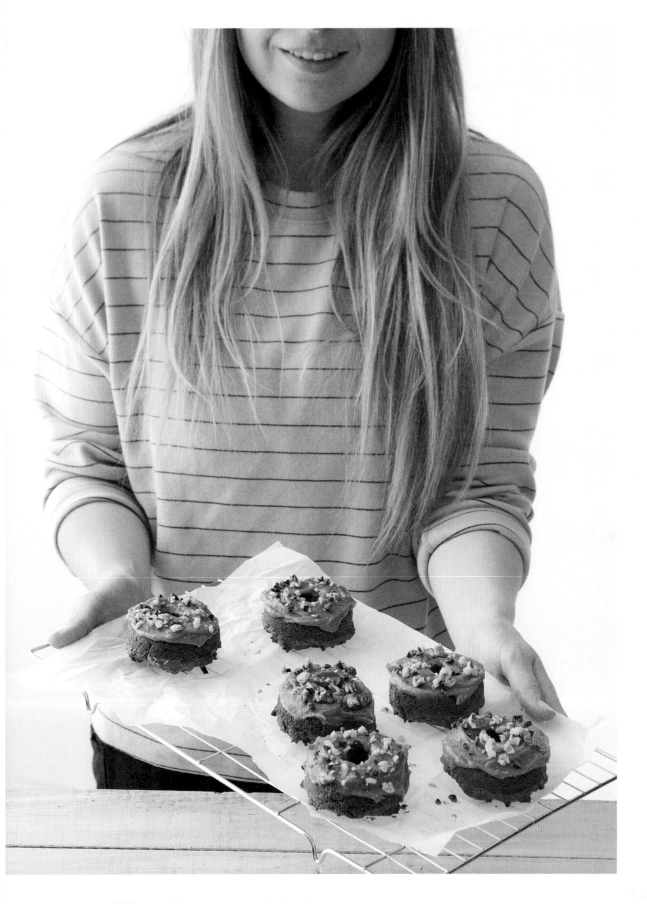

Breakfast

SMOOTHIES

Building the perfect hormone-balancing smoothie is all about finding a creamy, neutral base that complements the rest of the ingredients, as well as sufficiently nourishing your body. Strange though it may sound, cauliflower works brilliantly in this role, as does frozen sweet potato, courgette and avocado, all low in sugar to prevent blood sugar spikes. To this neutral base, add your fats and fibre – from nut butters to coconut oil, flaxseed to cacao nibs. These healthy sources will ensure you stay full and energised right up until lunchtime, as well as aiding in the production of healthy sex hormones.

Dose up on liver-loving B vitamins, including essential folate, by throwing in a handful of dark leafy greens. These will help kick-start the detoxification of used and counterproductive hormones through the liver, as well as giving you an anti-inflammatory boost.

CHOCOLATE ALMOND BUTTER SMOOTHIE

Serves 1

Prep: 15 minutes, plus overnight freezing

100 g (1 small) sweet potato (raw weight, before steaming and freezing)

250 ml (1 cup) almond milk (or any other plant-based milk)

1 tbsp raw cacao

1 tbsp almond butter

a handful of spinach

1 heaped tbsp maca powder

2 tbsp chia seeds or milled flaxseeds

1 scoop of high-quality plant-based protein (optional)

1 tbsp cacao nibs

1½ tbsp ashwagandha or 1½ tbsp chaga (optional)

1. Prepare the sweet potato the night before by peeling, chopping and steaming for about 10 minutes in a steamer basket. Transfer to the freezer overnight.
2. When you're ready to make your smoothie, throw all the ingredients into the blender and blend until completely smooth.

If you're worried about your protein intake on a plant-based diet, invest in a high-quality protein powder made using minimal ingredients. You can also add a couple of heaped tablespoons of hemp seeds, known to be the most easily digestible source of protein.

BLUEBERRY BREAKFAST SMOOTHIE

Serves 1

Prep: 5 minutes

250 ml (1 cup) almond milk

70 g (roughly ½ cup) frozen blueberries

150 g (5½ oz) frozen cauliflower florets (a large handful, roughly)

1 tbsp cashew nut butter

¼ tsp ground turmeric

½ tsp ground cinnamon (preferably Ceylon)

1–2 tbsp maca powder, depending on taste

2 tbsp rolled oats

a large handful of spinach

1 scoop of natural or vanilla plant-based protein powder (optional)

1. Place all the ingredients in a blender and blend until completely smooth and creamy.

Cinnamon is a fantastic addition to your morning smoothies as it is highly effective in regulating blood sugar, an essential part of any hormone-healthy diet. It is also highly anti-inflammatory and a potent antioxidant. If you find yourself consuming a large amount of cinnamon, ensure it's Ceylon, or 'true' cinnamon, as it is a purer source.

MINT CHOCOLATE CHIP SMOOTHIE

Serves 1

Prep: 5 minutes

250 ml (1 cup) plant-based milk

½ a frozen avocado

¼ a frozen banana

1 tbsp almond butter

a handful of spinach

a fistful of fresh mint

1 tbsp maca powder

1 tsp spirulina

1 scoop of hemp protein powder (optional)

1 tbsp cacao nibs

1. Place all the ingredients, with the exception of the cacao nibs, in a blender and blitz until completely smooth. Add the cacao nibs last, giving them a further blitz but ensuring they stay fairly whole.

JUICES

Too much fruit juice in one's diet, especially if you're in the process of creating balanced hormones through stabilising blood sugar levels, can actually be counterintuitive. When we juice, we take away the fibre and are left with the phytonutrients and sugar from the produce, which can spike blood sugar levels and irritate our adrenals, forcing insulin levels to over compensate and thus, throw things off balance. So, if your skin is playing up, your mood's a mess or you're holding onto excess weight in certain areas (all classic imbalance symptoms), then it is best to steer clear of juice cleanses.

However, juice is a fantastic tool when utilised in a way that supports the body, instead of working against it. Juicing up your green veggies is an excellent way of getting in those B vitamins and supporting the liver throughout its detoxification process; while carrot juice contains an amazing enzyme called amylase, which aids digestion and promotes healthy hormone detox pathways. Incorporating phytonutrient-rich vegetable juices into your diet is a great way of getting a quick boost. Here are a few of my favourites.

A juicer can be a fabulous tool to have in your kitchen. If you can, opt for a cold-press juicer, as these retain as many of the nutrients as possible without heating the juice, which can reduce the nutritional quality slightly.

SUNSHINE JUICE

Serves 2
Prep: 5 minutes
4 raw beetroots (roughly 500 g/1 lb 2 oz), plus the greens
2 oranges (roughly 300 g/10 1/2 oz)
4 medium-sized carrots
a thumb-sized piece of ginger

CELERY AND LIME JUICE

Serves 2
Prep: 5 minutes
500 g (1 lb 2 oz) celery
1 lime, peel removed

LIVER-SUPPORTING GREEN JUICE

Serves 2
Prep: 5 minutes
1 head of romaine lettuce
1 cucumber
2 large celery sticks
2 generous handfuls of spinach
1 lemon, peel removed
a thumb-sized piece of ginger
1 tsp spirulina

For all juices:
1. Wash all the ingredients before placing into a juicer.
2. Drink fresh.

Adaptogens in Smoothies

Adaptogens are herbs, often bought in powder form, that help
the body adapt to stress through nurturing the nervous system.
Since adding them into my diet, I have seen a tremendous
improvement in my physical PCOS symptoms and noticed
that a rather lovely 'come what may' outlook has magically
appeared into my life. Yes, most adaptogens taste absolutely
appalling – ashwagandha being the main culprit – however
they can be absolute game changers if you're feeling a little out
of whack. Add them to smoothies and hide the taste with rich
cacao, half a frozen banana or some ground cinnamon. While
they're definitely a lovely addition to a few recipes in this book,
they can be a little pricey and sometimes hard to find, so it's
completely up to you.

Celebrity Celery

Everyone needs to know about the incredible benefits that can
come from guzzling celery juice first thing in the morning.
Good gut health is the basis for, well, everything, and the
prebiotics in celery juice support healthy digestion from the
get-go by establishing a healthy environment. Alongside all the
wonderful phytonutrients, you'll also be getting a thoroughly
good cleanse of the liver.

From left to right: Sunshine Juice;
Celery and Lime Juice.

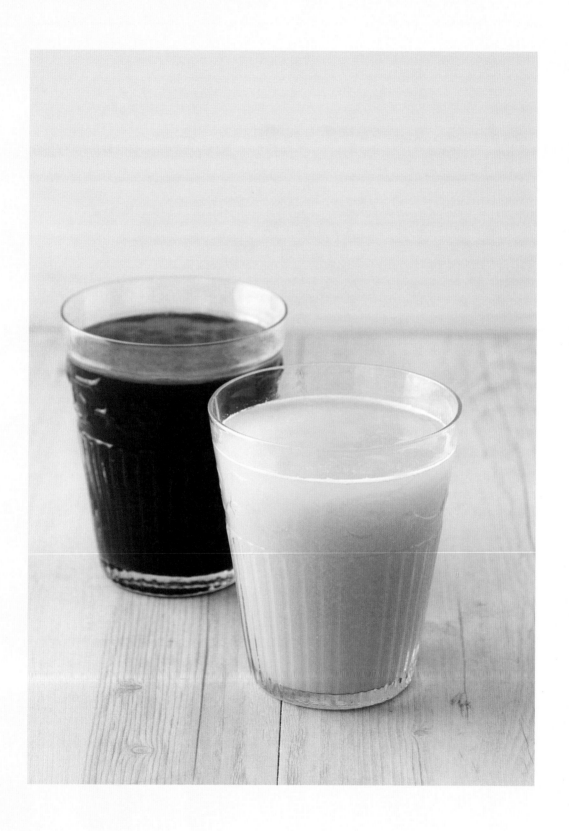

HOT MORNING ELIXIR

● ● ● ●

Hot lemon water has become the holy grail of the wellness world, and for a good reason. The combination of the two gives you a lovely wake up call first thing, with a dose of vitamin C from the lemon, promoting health progesterone production, and a digestive aid from the warm water itself. Let's take it up a notch with a lug of apple cider vinegar, amazing for fuelling your digestive fire, and by adding in a spoonful of ground cinnamon to balance blood sugar from the get-go. A grating of fresh ginger helps to keep seasonal illness at bay and is a great way to get in one of the most potent anti-inflammatory ingredients before the day has even begun.

Serves 1

Prep: 5 minutes

250 ml (1 cup) warm water
(boil and leave to cool)

1 tsp apple cider vinegar

½ tsp ground cinnamon
(preferably Ceylon)

¼ of a lemon, squeezed

a small piece of
ginger, grated

1. Place all the ingredients in a glass or mug, give it a good stir and sip slowly.

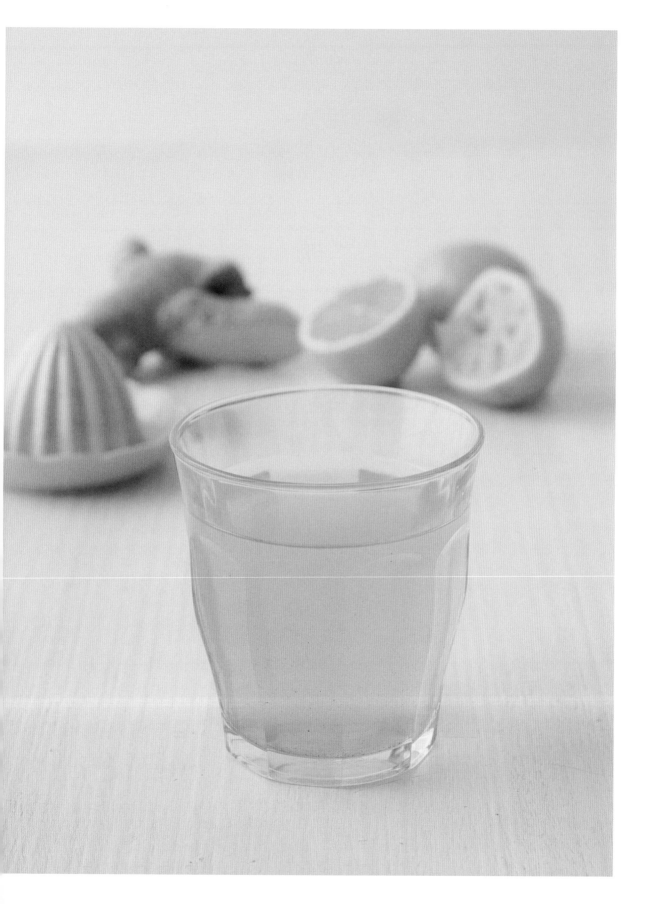

ALMOND BUTTER AND GINGER
CRUMBLE GRANOLA

● ● ● ●

In my childhood home sat a rhubarb plant and every year, once the stalks turned a vibrant pink colour, our house would transform into a crumble-making factory. I'd rub the butter and sugar between my fingers and dig out the stodgy section of pudding where the crumble met the gooey rhubarb as soon as it was out of the oven.

I'd pick at the cold leftovers for days to follow. A little bit here and there, even on occasion opting for a sneaky piece in place of breakfast. That is what inspired this recipe; a gorgeous ginger-spiced crumble granola that goes hand-in-hand with stewed rhubarb. An over generous helping of coconut yogurt acts the way custard would, and is the perfect finishing touch.

Makes 1 large jar

Prep: 10 minutes

Cook: 25 minutes

3 dates, stoned

3 tbsp smooth almond butter

2 tbsp coconut oil, melted

1 tbsp coconut sugar

300 g (3 cups) rolled oats

4 tbsp milled flaxseed

80 g (½ cup) flaked or chopped almonds

a large thumb-sized piece of ginger, grated

stewed rhubarb and a few generous dollops of dairy-free coconut yogurt, to serve

1. Preheat the oven to 180°C/350°F/gas mark 4.
2. Place the dates in a bowl of warm water and leave to soak for at least 10 minutes. Once soft, make a date caramel by blending the dates together with about 4 tablespoons of the soaking water, the almond butter, coconut oil and coconut sugar.
3. Add half the oats to the food processor, blending until broken up and combined with the date caramel. Place the mix into a large mixing bowl and add the remaining ingredients. Use your hands to ensure everything is well combined and that a crumbly yet sticky consistency is formed.
4. Place the crumbly granola mix on a lined baking tray, spreading out evenly. Bake for 25 minutes. Half way through give the oats a shuffle around with a wooden spoon, making sure everything gets an even bake. They should be golden brown with a slight crunch. Leave the granola to cool completely before transferring to a large glass jar.
5. Serve the granola with a side of stewed rhubarb (made by roughly chopping a few sticks and leaving them to simmer in a saucepan for 5 minutes with a splash of water) and a few generous dollops of coconut yogurt.

SPROUTED QUINOA PORRIDGE WITH
HAZELNUT BUTTER AND BLOOD ORANGE

● ● ● ●

I absolutely adore quinoa. Tossed into tumbles of roasted veg, baked into compact burger patties or as a trusty sidekick to creamy yellow dahl. So you can imagine it was quite the revelation when I first made sprouted quinoa porridge.

Aside from the fact that quinoa is incredibly versatile, it is also packed full of goodness. This gluten-free grain (actually a seed), is a fabulous plant-based protein source as well as containing all the essential amino acids. It's high in magnesium, a key mineral for balanced hormones as it helps to nurture fiery adrenal glands and improve insulin resistance.

Serves 2

Prep: 10 minutes, plus soaking overnight

Cook: 15 minutes

200 g (1 cup) quinoa (soaked overnight in cold water)

300 ml (1 ¼ cups) boiling water

200 ml (scant 1 cup) hazelnut milk (or any other plant-based milk of choice)

2 blood oranges, peeled and roughly chopped

1 tbsp hazelnut butter (or any other chosen fat source – I also like almond butter and coconut butter)

1 tbsp maple syrup (optional)

crushed roasted hazelnuts, to serve

1. Rinse the soaked quinoa thoroughly, then transfer to a saucepan with the boiling water over a low heat. It should take around 10 minutes for the quinoa to completely soak up all the water.
2. After 10 minutes, add the hazelnut milk and leave to simmer for a further 5 minutes. Keep an eye on it and stir every now and then to ensure it doesn't stick.
3. Meanwhile, place the peeled and chopped blood oranges into a second saucepan over a medium heat and leave to stew with a splash of water for 5 minutes.
4. Take both pans off the heat once your desired consistency is reached. Stir the hazelnut butter into the quinoa – you want to add some of these lovely fats to keep you fuller for longer and to nourish your body all day long.
5. Top with a drizzle of maple syrup, if you prefer a sweeter porridge. Sprinkle over the crushed hazelnuts and a generous spoonful of the stewed blood oranges.

I like to build my meals around seasonal produce as much as possible. Blood oranges come and go in a flash, but are absolutely gorgeous if you do get your hands on them. They are typically at their sweetest around the start of the year, when they are luxuriously dark and juicy. If you miss out, opt for your standard orange in this recipe, it's just as tasty – trust me!

SHORT-GRAIN BROWN RICE PORRIDGE WITH BAKED FIGS, SMASHED PISTACHIOS AND DAIRY-FREE COCONUT YOGURT

Porridge doesn't have to be made exclusively from oats and, in my opinion, there are many more exciting alternatives. While this version, made with short-grain brown rice, may take a little longer to cook, it's the most delicious and grounding way to start your day. I love the combination of gooey baked figs, sitting on top of thick coconut yogurt, finished with a fistful of smashed pistachio pieces. Dollop a spoonful of coconut butter in the centre and watch as it slowly melts to fill the bowl with a final puddle of natural sweetness. Three different high-fat ingredients mean you'll go about your day without any dreaded hunger pangs, full of energy and balanced blood sugar levels.

Serves 2

Prep: 10 minutes, plus soaking overnight

Cook: 45 minutes

100 g (½ cup) short-grain brown rice (soaked overnight in cold water)

500 ml (2 cups) boiling water

250 ml (1 cup) almond milk

a scraping of seeds from a vanilla pod, to taste

a pinch of ground cinnamon, to taste

TO TOP

2 fresh figs

maple syrup, for drizzling (optional)

1 tbsp coconut butter or almond butter if preferred

a dollop of dairy-free coconut yogurt

1 tbsp crushed pistachios

1. Preheat the oven to 200°C/400°F/gas mark 6.
1. Rinse the soaked short-grain brown rice thoroughly and place in a saucepan with the boiling water. Bring to the boil and continue to boil for 30 minutes, until the rice has soaked up all the water.
2. Slice the figs in half, place on a baking tray and bake for 15–20 minutes, until completely soft and gooey. Feel free to drizzle a little maple syrup over the top as they roast.
3. Once the brown rice has soaked up all the water, add the almond milk, vanilla seeds and cinnamon and leave to simmer for a further 15–20 minutes. This will line up perfectly with the cooking of the figs.
4. Keep stirring the porridge and add a touch more milk if you feel it needs it. When it's ready, spoon into a bowl, top with a spoonful of coconut butter, the coconut yogurt and crushed pistachios. Place the gooey figs on top to serve.

If you're prone to blood sugar spikes, or highly sensitive to sugar, then save the gooey figs for special occasions and swap for berries. Berries are lower in natural sugars and taste just as delicous.

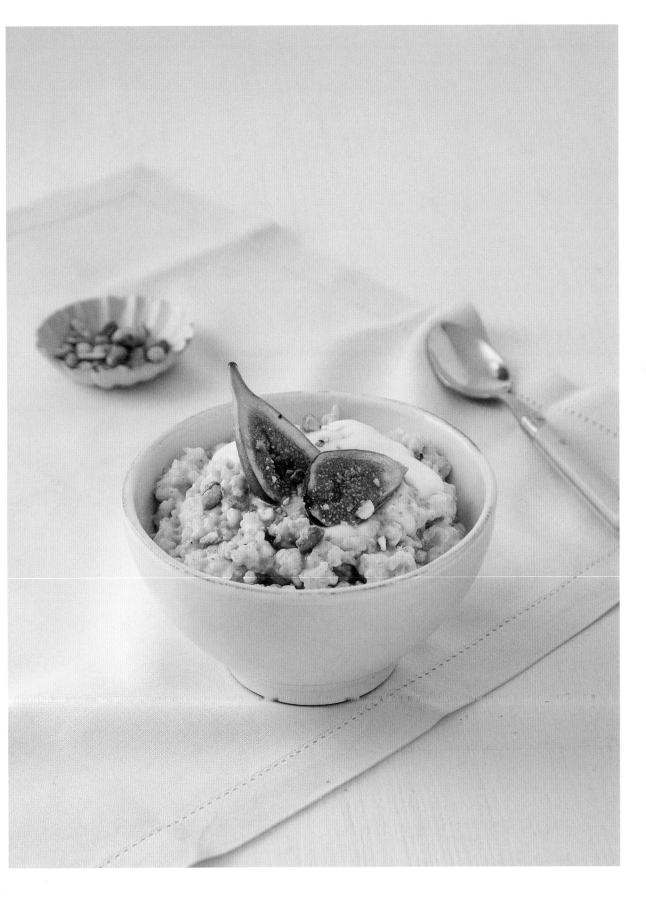

OVERNIGHT TEFF BREAKFAST BOWL WITH CHIA JAM

● ● ● ●

Teff — an Ethiopian grain — should be a staple in any hormone-healthy diet and it's subtle, delicate flavour makes it super versatile to cook with. From thick chocolate pancakes served with juicy cherries (Cherry Cacao Teff Pancakes, page 86), to this quick and easy, tummy happy, overnight porridge. It's high in iron, magnesium and zinc – all key nutrients for optimal hormone health. Teff is also known for being fibre rich, promoting a healthy, thriving environment in your gut, vital for a flourishing body and happy mind. Paired with high-fat probiotic coconut yogurt, this recipe will help banish any unwelcome bloat from slightly out of whack hormones, boost energy levels and the immune system, setting you up for whatever the day may throw at you.

Serves 1

Prep: 5 minutes, soaking overnight

120 ml (4 ½ oz) (roughly ½ cup) dairy-free coconut yogurt

50 g (¼ cup) teff grain

1 tbsp milled flaxseeds

½ tsp ground cinnamon (preferably Ceylon)

a fistful of fresh raspberries

½ tbsp chia seeds

1 tbsp nut butter of choice

1. Measure out the coconut yogurt in a bowl and add the teff, flaxseeds and cinnamon. Give everything a good mix before transferring into a jar to stand overnight.

2. The next morning, make a quick chia jam by mashing the raspberries together with the chia seeds and allowing to sit for five minutes. Spoon the jam onto the soaked teff, to serve, and finish with a generous spoonful of nut butter, if you wish.

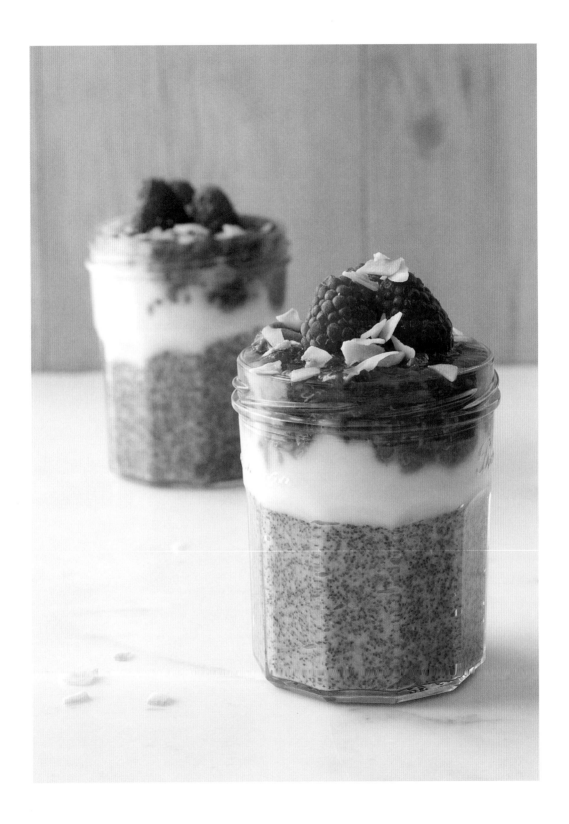

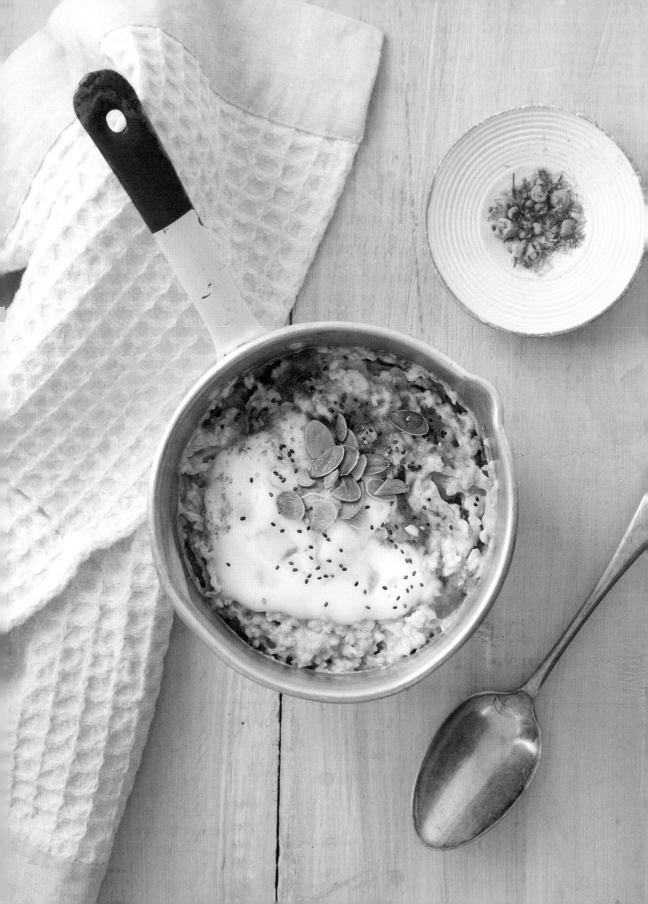

CAMOMILE AND MAPLE PORRIDGE

● ● ● ●

This recipe for camomile and maple porridge is my way of finding a moment of peace and serenity in the morning. Camomile is known as the ultimate soother, often drunk in hot tea at bedtime. However, there are no rules stating it can't be enjoyed at other times, and it is a lovely way of incorporating a bit of calm into your morning routine. Maple syrup has a deep and distinctive flavour, that works well against the muted floral taste of camomile. Top with flaked almonds and a spoonful of coconut butter for a sweet finish.

Serves 1

Prep: 5 minutes

Cook: 10 minutes

50 g (½ cup) rolled oats

100 ml (scant ½ cup) boiling water

230 ml (scant 1 cup) plant-based milk (I like to use cashew here)

2 tsp dried camomile flowers (or an emptied camomile tea bag)

TO TOP

1 tbsp coconut butter

1 tsp maple syrup

toasted flaked almonds
1 tbsp of flax seeds and/or chia seeds

1. Place the oats in a small saucepan over a low heat and pour in the boiling water and plant-based milk. Add the camomile flowers or tea leaves and mix until everything is combined. Cook for 10 minutes, stirring constantly.
2. You can fish out larger chunks of the flowers if you wish or leave them in. Simply serve with a spoonful of coconut butter on top, a drizzle of maple syrup, flaked almonds and a sprinkle of flax and chia seeds.

RASPBERRY AND COCONUT
BAKED AMARANTH PORRIDGE

● ● ● ●

This teeny tiny gluten-free grain, while a pain to clear up when spilt all over the kitchen worktop, is worth getting your hands on nonetheless. It's one of those pesky pseudograins which actually isn't a grain at all, and in fact, is a seed. Not only is amaranth gluten-free, it also contains all those lovely amino acids and is a great way to get in your plant-based protein. It's high in fibre, great for supporting a healthy gut and essential for the healthy detoxification of used hormones that no longer serve us.

This makes for a fabulous blow-out breakfast dish to serve warm or cold, topped with crunchy pumpkin seeds, toasted coconut flakes and a generous dollop of dairy-free coconut yogurt or nut butter to finish.

Serves 2

Prep: 10 minutes, plus soaking overnight

Cook: 50-60 minutes

200 g (1 cup) amaranth (soaked overnight in cold water)

400 ml (14 oz) can of full-fat coconut milk

½ tsp ground cinnamon (preferably Ceylon)

a scraping of seeds from a vanilla pod

1 tbsp milled flaxseed

a fistful of raspberries, fresh or frozen

a couple of tablespoons of toasted coconut flakes and pumpkin seeds, for topping

a dollop of your nut butter of choice and dairy-free coconut yogurt, to serve

1. Preheat the oven to around 200°C/400°F/gas mark 6.
1. Thoroughly rinse the soaked amaranth and place in a saucepan with the coconut milk, cinnamon and the scraped vanilla seeds. Leave to simmer gently for 20 minutes until all the coconut milk has been absorbed.
2. Place the flaxseed with 2 tablespoons water in a small bowl and leave to stand until the amaranth has cooked. It should go nice and gooey.
3. Pour the flaxseed into the pan once the amaranth has cooked and give it a good mix. Pour the amaranth into an ovenproof dish, so that the amaranth sits fairly thick. Press the raspberries into the mix and bake for 30–40 minutes.
4. With about 5 minutes to go, sprinkle the coconut flakes and pumpkin seeds on top and place back into the oven until the flakes go golden brown.
5. Leave to cool slightly, then serve with a dollop of nut butter and coconut yogurt.

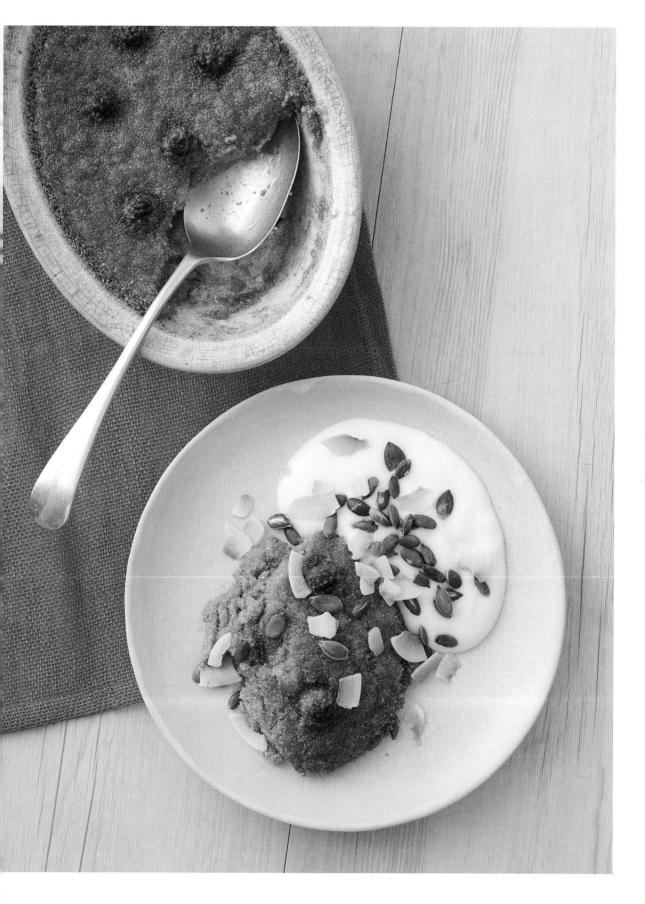

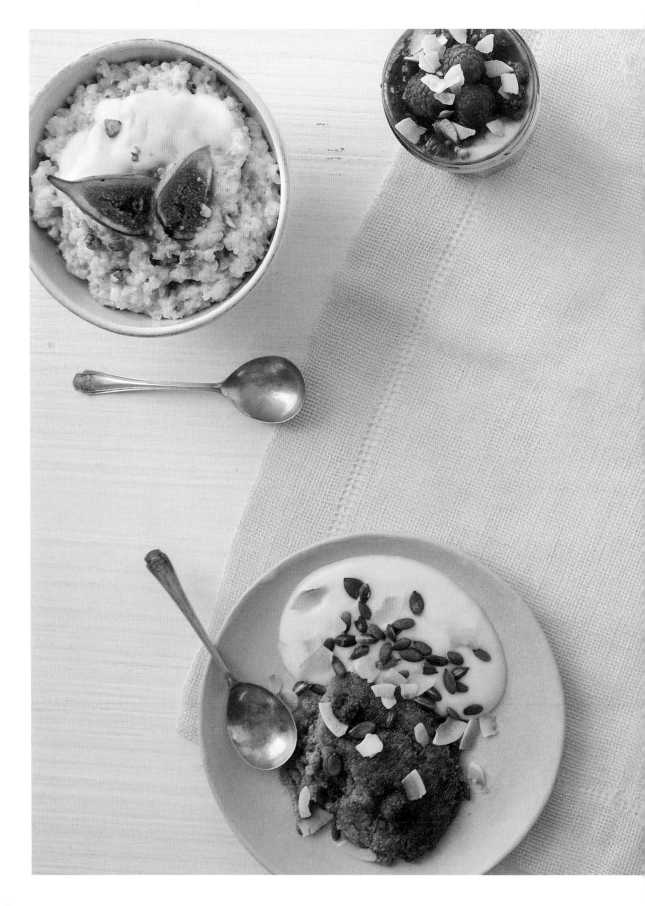

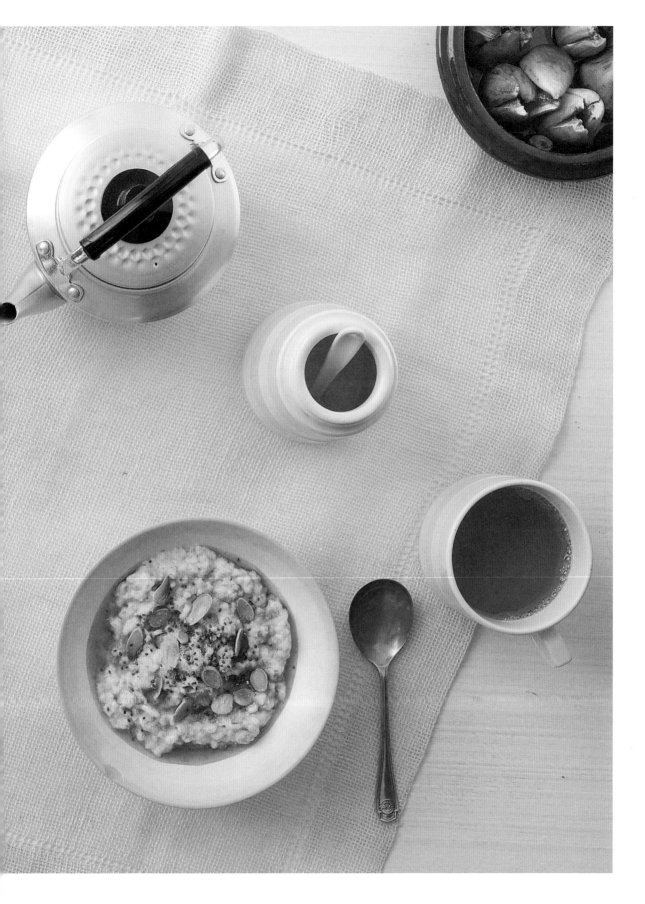

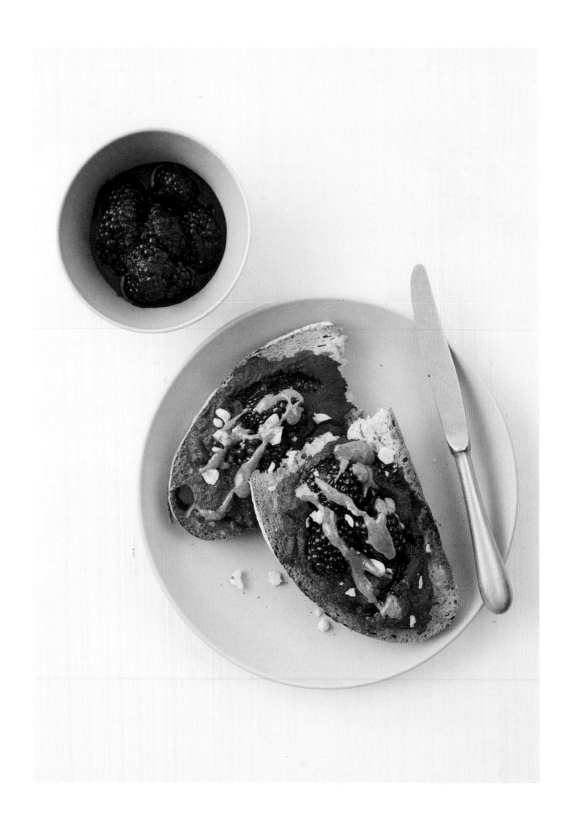

SWEET BEETROOT HUMMUS ON SOURDOUGH WITH BLACKBERRY JAM AND HAZELNUT BUTTER

● ● ● ●

I like my beetroot hummus vibrant and rich, that's why there is an obnoxious ratio of beetroot to chickpeas in this recipe. Embrace it! Beetroots are rich in folate (a fabulous fertility friendly vitamin), antioxidants and highly anti-inflammatory. Steamed and blended with chickpeas – an almighty source of plant-based protein – along with healthy fats found in both tahini and hazelnut butter, this super-spread will help stabilise unruly blood sugar levels.

Makes 1 large jar

Prep: 20 minutes

Cook: 25 minutes

280 g (10 oz) raw beetroot, peeled and chopped

400 g (14 oz) can of chickpeas, drained

1 tbsp tahini

1 tsp ground cumin

4 tbsp extra virgin olive oil

1 garlic clove

a squeeze of lemon juice

salt and black pepper

TO SERVE

toasted sourdough bread

a handful of blackberries, fresh or frozen

1 tbsp hazelnut butter or 2 tbsp roasted hazelnuts, smashed

1. To make the beetroot hummus, place the beetroot in a steamer basket and steam for about 20 minutes. Beets can be a bit of a pain to steam, so give them enough time to completely soften.

2. While the beets are steaming, rinse the chickpeas thoroughly and remove the skins. You can do this by gently pinching the edge and letting the chickpea pop out. This will make for an extra smooth hummus.

3. Place the peeled chickpeas and the soft beetroots into a food processor or blender along with the rest of the hummus ingredients. Blend for a good few minutes until completely smooth.

4. Toast the bread and place the blackberries in a saucepan over a medium heat with a touch of water. Leave to stew for 5 minutes.

5. Spread the beetroot hummus generously on the toast, pile on the stewed blackberries and drizzle over the hazelnut butter or smashed nuts to finish.

STRAWBERRIES AND AVOCADO ON SOURDOUGH ● ● ● ●

I can only apologise that you're a few pages of recipes into the book, and already you've come across avocado toast. I do promise you, however, that this is a good one. Avocado on toast is the kind of food you can whip up within a matter of moments for guests staying the night, or simply as a mid-morning snack. I'll top mine with strawberries and a drizzle of balsamic to liven things up a bit and add a hint of unexpected sweetness against the greatness that is creamy smashed avocado.

Serves 2

Prep: 5 minutes

Cook: 3 minutes

2 slices of good quality bread (sourdough, gluten-free – your choice)

1 ripe avocado

1 tsp olive oil

a squeeze of lime juice

200 g (7 oz) strawberries, tops removed and sliced

a drizzle of balsamic vinegar (optional)

a fistful of hulled hemp seeds and pumpkin seeds

salt and black pepper

1. Toast the bread and slice your avocado down the centre, removing the stone. Chop up the flesh into chunks before placing in a small bowl with the olive oil and squeeze of lime juice, mashing it all together with a spoon.
2. Pile the smashed avocado up on your toast and season generously. Top with sliced strawberries, a drizzle of balsamic vinegar and some hemp and pumpkin seeds.

Let's Talk About Bread

Bread is an interesting one and can sometimes get a bit of a bad rep when it comes to health. However, you can absolutely incorporate it into a healthy, balanced diet. Opt for minimal ingredients when choosing your loaf and choose wholegrain, which is packed full of seeds for a slower release of energy and fibre hit, or sourdough, which is kinder on digestion.

Dairy-free Coconut Yogurt

I eat dairy-free coconut yogurt every single day as it is so wonderfully nourishing. Pick up a pot that has minimal ingredients and no added sugar for an easy on-the-go snack, or even as a great way to freshen up curries, soups and dahls.

CHERRY CACAO TEFF PANCAKES

● ● ● ●

These thick, fluffy and wholesome cherry cacao pancakes are Sunday brunch food at its finest, and another easy way to incorporate teff, one of my favourite hormone-healthy ingredients, into your life. Pile a few generously overflowing spoonfuls of sweet stewed cherries on top of your chocolate stack, or tip straight into the mix itself, the combination of the two flavours really is as good as it sounds. This recipe is the perfect example of how you can make those really-good-for-you foods that you know you probably should eat, into meals you actually really want to eat.

Serves 2
Prep: 10 minutes
Cook: 10 minutes

1 tbsp milled flaxseed

60 g (2¼ oz) rolled oats

1 ripe banana

60 g (2¼ oz) teff flour

130 ml (½ cup) almond milk

2 tbsp cacao powder

½ tsp baking powder

a touch of coconut oil, for frying

150 g (5½ oz) fresh or frozen cherries, stoned

dairy-free coconut yogurt, nut butter and/ or maple syrup to serve

1. Place the flaxseed in a small bowl with 2 tablespoons water and leave to thicken while you complete the next step.
2. Place the rolled oats into a food processor or blender and blitz until a fine flour forms. Add in all the remaining ingredients, with the exception of the coconut oil and cherries, and blend for a short moment until combined. Add the soaked flaxseeds and stir in by hand.
3. Pop a frying pan over a low heat with a touch of coconut oil and roughly 60 ml (¼ cup) sized amounts of the batter into the pan. Dot a couple of the frozen or chopped fresh cherries into the mix, if you wish.
4. Leave to cook for 5 minutes or so on each side. You'll want to keep the heat fairly low to avoid burning the surface and to cook the middle fully.
5. Cook the remaining cherries in a saucepan with a touch of water and leave to completely soften before serving on top of the pancakes. Finish with coconut yogurt, nut butter, maple syrup – whatever you like.

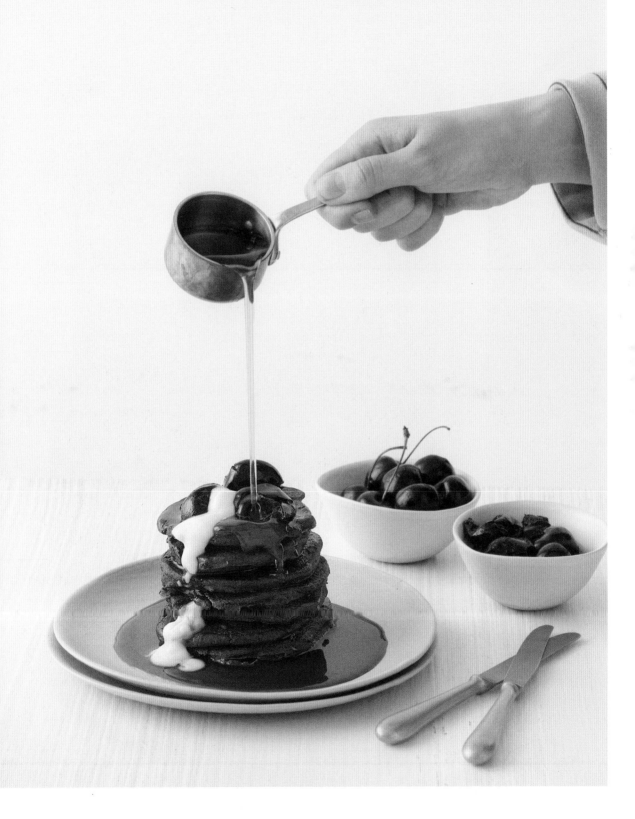

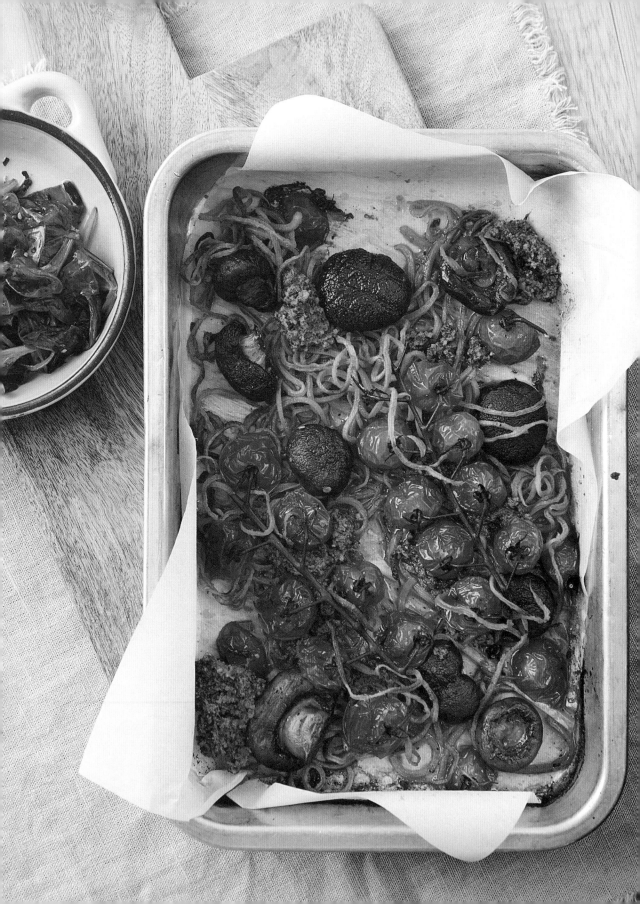

VEGGIE BREAKFAST TRAY BAKE

● ● ● ● ●

While pancake stacks and sweet bowls of filling porridge are all well and good, there is a lot to be said for a decent full English veggie breakfast. The kind of veggie breakfast where each individual component really holds its own and is full of flavour and sustenance. Slow-roasted vine tomatoes, doused in rich olive oil, really are as glorious as they sound, and become ever so soft and juicy when cooked in this way. Eat them alongside crispy tangles of sweet potato for an easy alternative to hash browns, and a creamy side of sliced avocado – a savoury brunch superhero if there ever was one.

Serves 2

Prep: 10 minutes

Cook: 30 minutes

240 g (8 ½ oz) cherry tomatoes (ideally still on the vine)

200 g (7 oz) chestnut mushrooms

a generous drizzle of extra virgin olive oil

2 small sweet potatoes (about 130 g/4 oz each)

a sprinkle of dried chilli flakes

2 tsp Brazil Nut Pesto (see page 182)

1 garlic clove, minced

2 generous handfuls of spinach

1 ripe avocado, peeled, stoned and sliced

2 tbsp Homemade Hummus (see page 188)

salt and black pepper

1. Preheat the oven to 180°C/350°F/gas mark 4. Line your baking tray with a sheet of baking parchment.
2. Place the cherry tomatoes and whole chestnut mushrooms on a large baking tray with a generous drizzle of olive oil and season with salt and pepper. Bake for 10 minutes.
3. Cut the sweet potatoes lengthways, so that they are thin enough to fit into your spiraliser with ease. Spiralise them, then toss the potato noodles with a touch of olive oil and some chilli flakes before placing on the tray with the tomatoes and mushrooms. Cook everything for a further 20 minutes.
4. With roughly 5 minutes to go, add a dollop of pesto on top of the tomatoes, and heat a medium pan with a drizzle of olive oil. Add the garlic and spinach to the pan, allowing it to completely wilt down. Plate up all the cooked components and finish with a side of sliced avocado and a dollop of hummus.

Lunch & Dinner

ROASTED CARROT, PEARLED SPELT AND ORANGE SALAD

● ● ● ●

I'm a huge advocate for soaking your grains, seeds and nuts. Mostly because doing so takes a little pressure off the busy body that is your digestive system. Soaking also aids the breakdown of phytic acid, which can mess around with the absorption of minerals in the body, such as zinc. We want to grab hold of the zinc in our bodies for dear life, as it's a key mineral for hormonal balance and especially essential if you're having issues with your skin. For this recipe, soak your spelt overnight ready to eat the following evening.

Perfect eaten warm, this salad also keeps well in the fridge for a couple of days, so save those leftovers for weekday lunches.

Serves 2 as a main, 4 as a side

Prep: 10 minutes plus soaking overnight

Cook: about 30 minutes

1 red onion, chopped

300 g (10 ½ oz) baby carrots, greens in tact

2 tbsp extra virgin olive oil, plus extra for drizzling

200 g (1 cup) dry spelt (soaked overnight in cold water)

1 medium orange

2 generous handfuls of kale, finely shredded

2 tbsp apple cider vinegar

6 whole dried figs, finely chopped

a fistful of crushed roasted hazelnuts

sea salt and cracked black pepper

1. Preheat the oven to 200 °C/400 °F/gas mark 6.
2. Place the red onion on a baking tray with the carrots (greens removed and set aside) and a drizzle of olive oil. Season with salt and pepper and roast for 20 minutes.
3. Once the carrots and red onion have gone into the oven, thoroughly rinse the soaked spelt and boil over a medium heat for 20 minutes as well.
4. Grate the zest from the orange and set aside. Squeeze the juice from the orange.
5. Place the shredded kale in a large bowl along with the 2 tbsp of olive oil, apple cider vinegar and orange juice, massaging it into the kale for 5 minutes.
6. Add the cooked spelt, roasted carrots and onion and carrot greens to the bowl with the kale.
7. Toss in the orange zest, finely chopped dried figs and crushed hazelnuts. Give everything a good mix and feel free to season further with cracked black pepper and sea salt, before drizzling with a little extra olive oil.

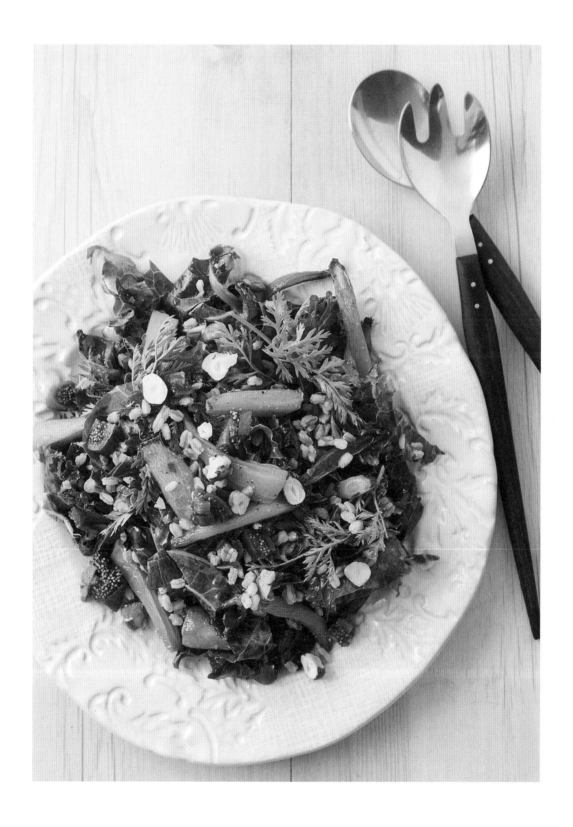

ROASTED FENNEL, ROCKET AND WILD RICE SALAD WITH BROCCOLI CREAM

● ● ● ●

If you're not a fennel fan, you've obviously never tried roasting it. After sitting in the oven for 30 minutes (at least), seasoned with sea salt flakes and cracked black pepper, the fennel becomes gooey and soft in between the layers and slightly crisp around the edges. It's a real treat.

From a health perspective, this delicious salad is a game changer. Broccoli sprouts are optional, as they can be tricky to get your hands on, however they are definitely worth mentioning as a hormone-balancing superhero ingredient to toss into salads. They contain sulforaphane, a fantastic compound that supports your liver through its natural detoxification process thus rebalancing oestrogen levels.

Serves 4

Prep: 10 minutes, plus soaking overnight

Cook: 50 minutes

250 g (1½ cups) wild rice (soaked overnight in cold water, ideally)

2 medium fennel bulbs, plus the fennel fronds

avocado oil, for cooking

25 g (1 oz) pumpkin seeds

25 g (1 oz) sunflower seeds

150 g (5½ oz) green beans

2 large handfuls of rocket

50 g (1¾ oz) broccoli sprouts (optional)

BROCCOLI CREAM

45 g (¼ cup) cashews (soaked for at least 30 minutes in cold water)

100 g (3½ oz) broccoli

2 tbsp nutritional yeast

4 tbsp extra virgin olive oil

a squeeze of lemon juice

salt and cracked black pepper

1. Preheat the oven to 200°C/400°F/gas mark 6. Rinse the soaked rice thoroughly, transfer to a saucepan of water to cover, and boil for 40 minutes.

2. Once the rice is cooking, slice the fennel vertically into quarters, allowing the layers to still hold together. Keep the fennel fronds to the side. Place on a baking tray with a generous drizzle of avocado oil and a sprinkle of salt and black pepper. Bake for 30 minutes at least, until it softens and the edges start to brown.

3. With about 15 minutes to go until your rice and fennel are cooked, toast the seeds for a couple of minutes in a dry pan and set aside until ready to serve. Place the green beans in a griddle pan with a touch of oil and leave to cook for about 5 minutes.

4. To make the broccoli cream, steam the broccoli in a steamer basket for 5 minutes until soft. Add the soft broccoli and all the remaining broccoli cream ingredients to a blender and blend until completely smooth. Add a splash of water to help reach a creamy consistency.

5. Drain the wild rice, placing it in a large sharing bowl with the roasted fennel, grilled green beans and couple of generous handfuls of rocket. Toss everything together. Throw in the broccoli sprouts, if using, and sprinkle over the toasted seeds. Add dollops of the broccoli cream around the corners of the large sharing bowl, or serve in a small pot on the side.

GRILLED COURGETTE, ASPARAGUS AND ROCKET SALAD

There is nothing worse than badly cooked courgettes. The kind that is part soggy, part crunchy, and always ends up looking a little sad on your plate. No wonder those lovely greens get a bit of a bad rep sometimes, we simply aren't giving them enough love. One of my favourite ways to eat courgettes, is to slice them lengthways into thin ribbons and grill them with a lug of olive oil, salt and pepper. I'll then toss the chargrilled strips, complete with beautiful black grill marks, onto a bed of fresh rocket, jumbled among asparagus spears, creamy avocado slices and finish with a drizzle of homemade pesto.

**Serves 2 as a main,
4 as a side**
Prep: 10 minutes
Cook: 10 minutes

2 large courgettes, washed
avocado oil, for frying
200 g (7 oz) asparagus
2 large handfuls of rocket
2 tbsp Coriander
Pesto (see page 182)
1 large ripe avocado
a grating of lemon zest
a drizzle of extra
virgin olive oil
salt and black pepper
a fistful of toasted
seeds, to garnish

1. Remove the top and ends of the courgettes and slice lengthways into 5 mm (¼ in) ribbons. Heat up a griddle pan with a touch of oil and place each courgette strip on to cook for 5 minutes, flipping halfway to ensure an even cook.

2. Meanwhile, prepare a steamer basket, add the asparagus and cook for roughly 3–4 minutes, until you can easily stick a fork through. Once cooked, toss together with the rocket and a generous spoonful of pesto.

3. Lay over the grilled courgettes and slice the ripe avocado, placing on top of the rest of the salad. Season with a crack of black pepper and salt, lemon zest and a drizzle of extra virgin olive oil, to finish. I throw a fistful of toasted seeds over my salads at the final stage, for some added texture.

Looking for something a bit more filling?
Cook up a batch of quinoa or buckwheat and toss
it in with the veggies.

DELICATA SQUASH AND BLACK RICE
SALAD WITH BRAZIL NUT PESTO

Another glorious salad, this time championing gooey, caramelised squash. Delicata squash, with its wonderfully scalloped skin and sweet taste, is the real star of this show. However, the humble butternut squash also works well here. Pair with antioxidant-rich black rice and you have yourself a cosy autumnal salad, eaten warm and shared among friends on chilly evenings, or taken to work as a fancy packed lunch. These types of recipes make eating well an absolute breeze, as it's the type of meal you can slowly pull together and leave to cook away on its own.

Serves 4

Prep: 10 minutes, plus soaking overnight

Cook: 40 minutes

1 large delicata or butternut squash

avocado oil for cooking

180 g (1 cup) black rice (soaked overnight)

1 red onion, sliced

250 g (9 oz) raw beetroot, chopped, greens in tact

1 garlic clove, minced

a few generous handfuls of leafy greens, chopped (I like cavolo nero for this recipe, but rocket and chard also work well)

2 tbsp Brazil Nut Pesto (see page 182)

a handful of crushed roasted hazelnuts

salt and black pepper

Quick and Simple Hummus (see page 188), to serve

1. Preheat the oven to 200°C/400°F/gas mark 6. Slice the top and bottom off the squash before cutting lengthways. Scoop out the seeds and cut into crescent-shaped chunks. Place on a baking tray with a generous drizzle of avocado oil and salt and pepper. Bake for 40 minutes until golden brown and soft.

2. Meanwhile, thoroughly wash the soaked rice, transfer to a large saucepan and cover with boiling water. Boil for 40 minutes, until lovely and chewy.

3. With 30 minutes to go, slice the onion and chop the beetroots (setting the greens aside) and put on another baking tray, seasoned well and drizzled with a touch of oil. Roast for 30 minutes.

4. One the rice is cooked, heat a second large pan, add a lug of oil and throw in the garlic, leafy greens and beetroot greens to cook down. Add the drained rice and pesto, thoroughly mixing everything before tipping out into a large bowl.

5. Add the roasted veg and crushed hazelnuts and toss everything together. Serve with a side of homemade hummus.

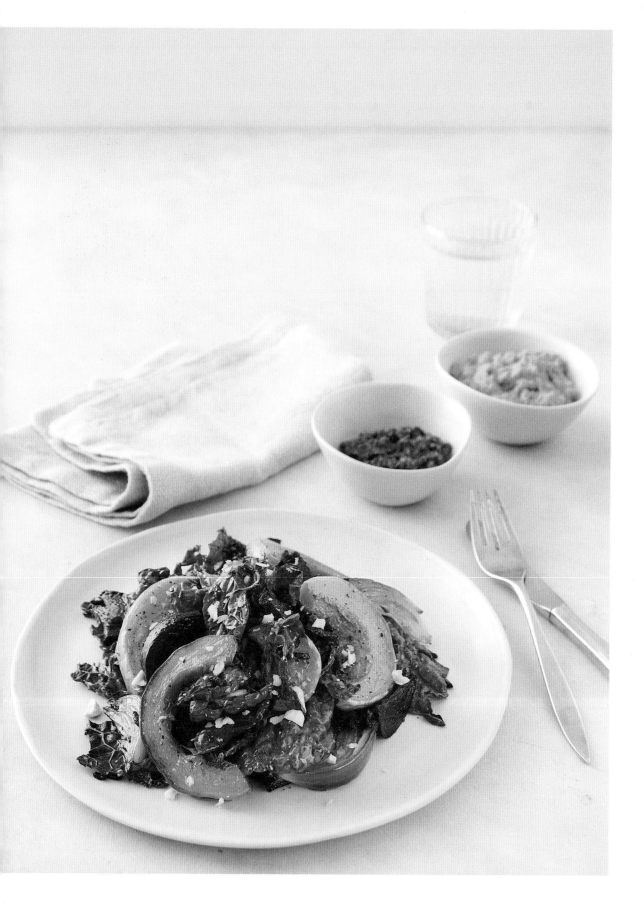

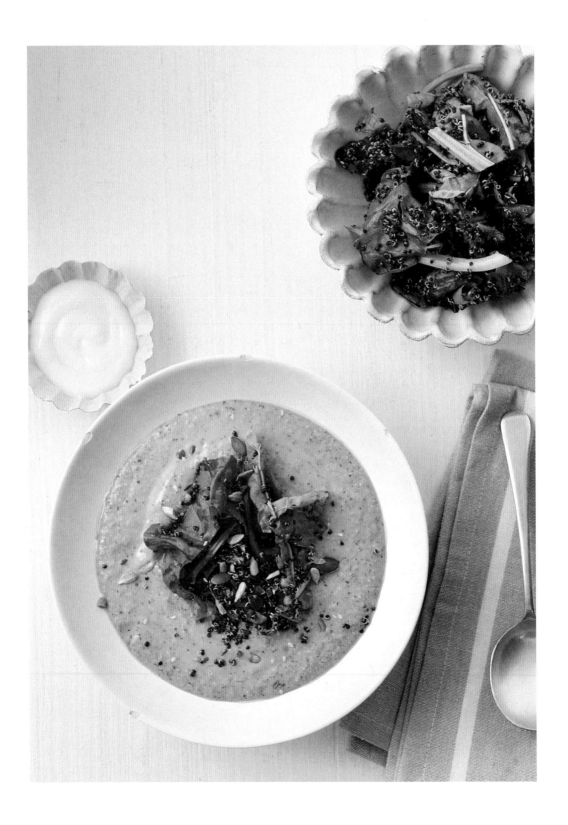

CHILLED AVOCADO AND PEA SOUP
WITH BLACK QUINOA

● ● ● ●

A wonderful medley of springtime flavours, this chilled avocado and pea soup is refreshing and indulgently creamy. The star of the show, avocado, is rich in folate, mood-boosting and one of the best ways you can pack in those monounsaturated fats. Serve as a light, fresh starter or pair with quinoa and leafy greens, such as cavolo nero, for a more substantial main. In the colder months, serve warm with a dollop of coconut yogurt for a comforting alternative.

Serves 2

Prep: 10 minutes, plus 4 hours soaking

Cook: 20 minutes

250 g (2 cups) fresh or frozen peas

1 large ripe avocado (about 215 g/7½ oz)

6 fresh mint leaves

40 g (¼ cup) cashews, (soaked for at least 4 hours in cold water)

a squeeze of lemon juice

2 tbsp nutritional yeast

130 g (scant 1 cup) quinoa

a generous handful of chopped leafy greens

salt and black pepper

TO SERVE

15 g (½ oz) pumpkin seeds

15 g (½ oz) sunflower seeds

2 tbsp hemp seeds

a dollop of dairy-free coconut yogurt

1. Place the peas in a saucepan over a low heat with a splash of water and cook for about 5 minutes. Once cooked, transfer to a food processor or blender and add the avocado, mint leaves, soaked cashews, lemon juice, nutritional yeast and 500 ml (2 cups) water. Blend until completely smooth and creamy before placing in the fridge to chill for an hour or so.
2. Boil the quinoa in 500 ml (2 cups) of water for about 15 minutes in a pan over a medium heat and allow all the water to be absorbed.
3. Once cooked, add the chopped leafy greens to the quinoa and allow to wilt over a low heat. Gently toast the seeds ready to serve.
4. Leave the quinoa to cool and divide between two bowls, gently pouring the soup over. Top with the seeds and coconut yogurt.

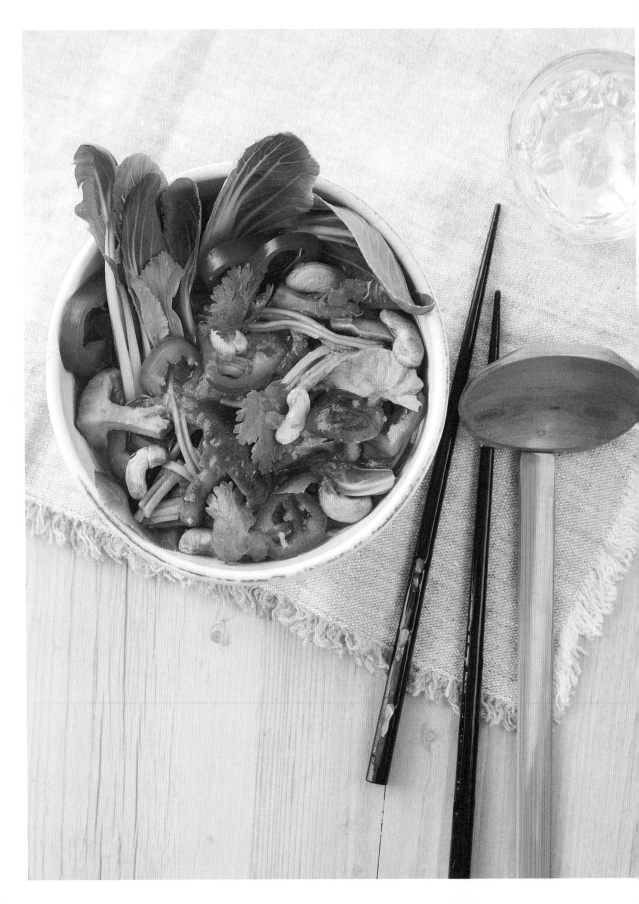

HEALING SHIITAKE MUSHROOM MISO SOUP WITH BUCKWHEAT SOBA NOODLES

● ● ● ●

A day or two post-Christmas feasting, my Dad always makes his veggie-packed miso soup. Trust me, this recipe is a god-send once the festivities have died down. Complete with chewy buckwheat noodles, leafy greens and a generous grating of fresh ginger, this soup is everything you could possibly ask for. It's light on the digestive system and highly anti-inflammatory, making it a must have for when you're not quite feeling yourself. From nursing Christmas dinner food babies, to curing painful hormonal migraines, it's a hug in a bowl, to say the least.

Serves 2

Prep: 10 minutes

Cook: about 30 minutes

avocado or coconut
oil, for cooking

1 red onion, finely
chopped

2 garlic cloves, minced

125 g (4½ oz)
shiitake mushrooms,
roughly chopped

1 litre (4 cups)
boiling water

150 g (5½ oz) buckwheat
soba noodles

1 medium red Romano
pepper, sliced into rings

2 tbsp dark brown
rice miso paste

2 tbsp dried wakame
flakes or kombu

a generous handful of
choi sum, pak choi leaves
or any leafy greens

a thumb-sized piece of
ginger, peeled and grated

a pinch of dried chilli
flakes or chopped
fresh chilli, to taste

a fistful of lightly
toasted cashews

a fistful of fresh
coriander, chopped

1. Add a dash of oil to a large saucepan over a low to medium heat and add the finely chopped red onion. Leave to soften and brown ever so slightly before adding the garlic and mushrooms. Cook for 5 minutes.
2. Carefully pour in the boiling water and leave to simmer away for 20 minutes.
3. During this time, place the soba noodles in a bowl of boiling water to soften, or cook as per pack instructions.
4. When the 20 minutes is up, throw in the Romano pepper, miso paste and wakame or kombu and cook for 5 minutes. Ensure the pepper has softened before adding the greens and ginger.
5. At the very last moment, drain the soft buckwheat soba noodles and add to the soup. Serve with the chilli flakes, toasted cashews and coriander.

CHUNKY VEGGIE AND QUINOA SOUP

● ● ● ●

When the weather is bitter and sickness is quietly lurking, only one meal will suffice. Soup. Soup crammed full of chunky vegetables and wholesome grains, to be precise. The kind of meal you don't want to slave away over, chopping and gathering numerous different components, but instead, leave to simmer and do it's own thing. In this recipe, the carrots soften and the quinoa soaks up all of the flavour as it becomes wonderfully fluffy. A generous handful of earthy wild mushrooms, cooked simply in avocado oil and thyme is the perfect addition to an already great meal for chilly days. Drop a fistful of roasted seeds and chopped parsley on top and curl up with a blanket as you slurp the evening away.

Serves 2

Prep: 15 minutes

Cook: about 40 minutes

1 red onion, finely chopped

1 large celery stick, finely chopped

avocado oil, for cooking

2 garlic cloves, minced

2 medium carrots, roughly chopped

1½ litres (6 cups) boiling water

1 tsp ground turmeric

a fistful of dried porcini mushrooms

100 g (3½ oz) quinoa

a generous handful of kale

¼ head of white cabbage, sliced

100 g (3½ oz) wild mushrooms (I like chanterelles)

a fistful of thyme

a fistful of parsley

chopped and toasted pumpkin or sunflower seeds, to garnish

salt and black pepper

1. Place the red onion and celery in a large saucepan with a dash of avocado oil. Add the garlic and leave to cook down for 5 minutes. Throw in the carrots and gently pour in the boiling water. Add the turmeric and dried porcini mushrooms before leaving the soup to simmer for 15 minutes.

2. Add the quinoa, kale and sliced cabbage, leaving to cook for a further 15 minutes, until the quinoa has had some time to fluff up slightly.

3. In a separate pan, just before the soup has finished simmering, add a lug of avocado oil and throw in the wild mushrooms and thyme, cooking for a good few minutes until they catch a slight colour.

4. Serve in bowls, topped with the wild thyme mushrooms, fresh parsley and toasted seeds.

Want something a little heartier? Swap the quinoa for pearled barley. It'll take slightly longer to cook, roughly 30 minutes, but has a gloriously chewy texture that works perfectly here.

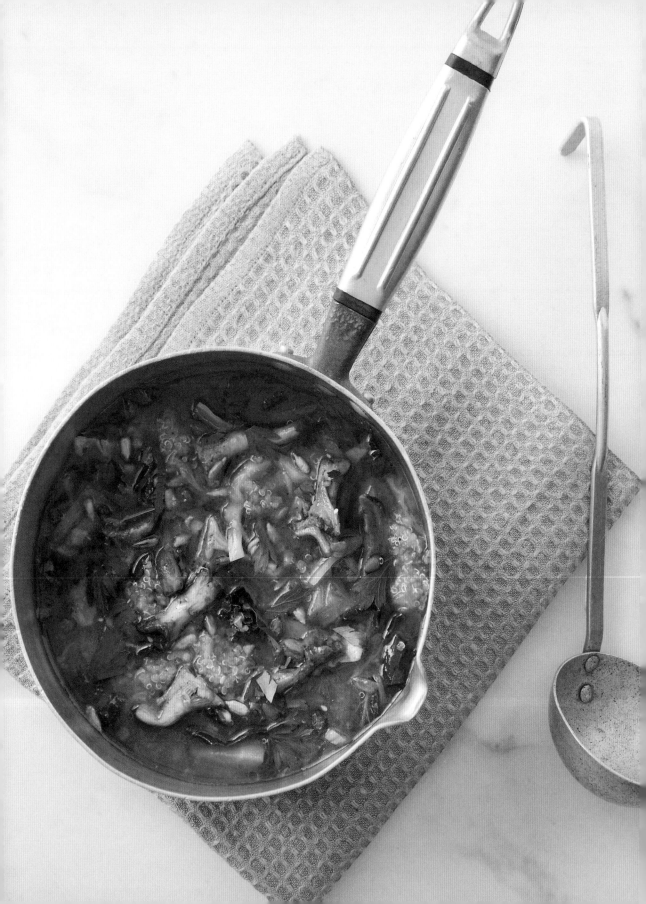

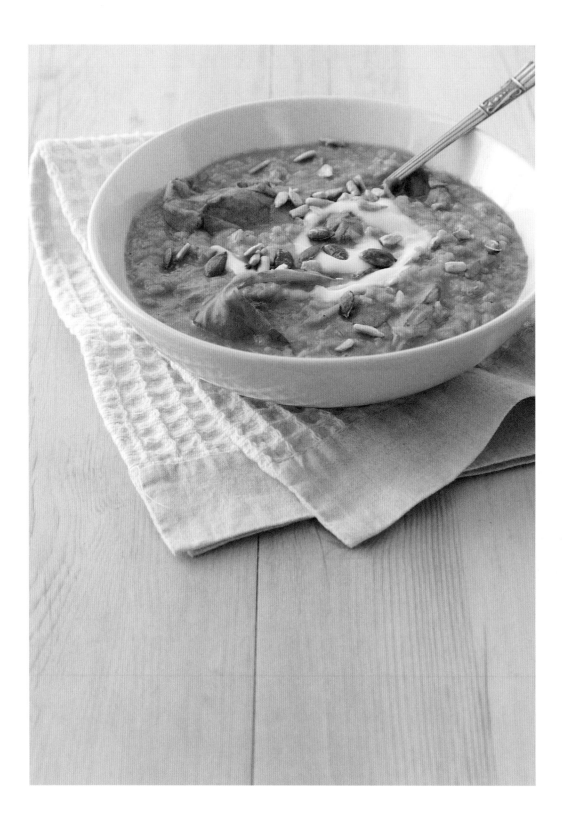

YELLOW AYURVEDIC DAHL WITH
SEASONAL GREENS

● ● ● ●

This is the meal I could, and almost do, eat every single day. It's easy, delicious and crammed full of the most nourishing, hormone-balancing ingredients you can get your hands on. From the incredible anti-inflammatory properties of turmeric and ginger, to protein-packed red lentils, dahl is a staple in ayurvedic diets due to its warming and wonderfully grounding properties. I add a whole can of full-fat coconut milk (apart from the thick cream on the top) because, well, I'm hoping you know by now just how great those fat-rich ingredients are for your body, and also chuck in a generous helping of liver-supporting leafy greens to wilt down at the last moment.

Serves 2

Prep: 10 minutes

Cook: 20–25 minutes

1 red onion, finely chopped

avocado oil or coconut oil, for cooking

1 garlic clove, minced

1 tsp ground turmeric

½ tsp ground fenugreek

½ tsp ground cinnamon

½ tsp fennel seeds

230 g (1½ cups) red lentils

400 ml (14 oz) can full-fat coconut milk (thick cream on top removed)

1 kaffir lime leaf

a thumb-sized piece of ginger, grated

700 ml (3 cups) boiling water (or enough to cover)

2 tbsp nutritional yeast (optional)

a couple of large handfuls of seasonal leafy greens, chopped (see Tip)

salt and black pepper

1. Place the red onion in a large pan with a dash of oil over a medium heat. Fry until browned slightly before adding the garlic.
2. In the corner of the pan, cook the spices with a touch more oil and then mix in with the onion.
3. Add the red lentils along with the coconut milk (the main bulk of thick cream resting on top should be removed and the liquid stirred before adding). Add the kaffir lime leaf, grated ginger and boiling water.
4. Simmer for 20 minutes over a medium heat, stirring continuously. The lentils should be completely soft and gloopy, if not, feel free to cook for longer. Just before serving, add the nutritional yeast, season generously with salt and pepper and mix in the chopped leafy greens.

My favourite greens are rainbow chard, cavolo nero or even just simple spinach. I'll often sneak greens into stews and dahl, piled on top of fluffy quinoa, finished with chopped coriander, a dollop of dairy-free coconut yogurt and a sprinkling of pumpkin seeds.

FLUFFY KITCHARI

● ● ● ●

I was making this recipe for years before I had any clue what it actually was. I'd throw wholegrain rice and red lentils into a pan with some water and let them bubble away until soft and gooey, sometimes even a little fluffy. Little did I know my standard university dinner was actually a take on an ayurvedic staple.

Nowadays, I keep the red lentils for creamy bowls of dahl, swapping mung beans in their place – the base of a classic Kitchari. Kitchari is a great way to give the digestive system a rest and feed the body vital nutrients and balancing spices.

Serves 1

Prep: 10 minutes, plus soaking overnight

Cook: 45 minutes

70 g (½ cup) split mung beans (soaked overnight)

45 g (½ cup) wild rice or brown basmati (soaked overnight in cold water)

700 ml (3 cups) boiling water

1 medium carrot

a generous handful of kale, chopped and stems removed

1 tbsp coconut oil

½ tsp ground turmeric

½ tsp ground fenugreek

½ tsp fennel seeds

a thumb-sized piece of ginger

salt and black pepper

fresh coriander, chopped and a heaped tablespoon of dairy-free coconut yogurt, to serve

1. Make sure the soaked beans have split slightly, then rinse thoroughly and set aside.
2. Place the rice and mung beans in a saucepan over a medium heat along with the boiling water and simmer for 40 minutes. With about 5 minutes to go, grate in the carrot and add the chopped kale. Reduce the heat and cover with a lid and cook gently until all the liquid is absorbed.
3. Melt the coconut oil in a saucepan over a low heat and leave to completely melt. Add the turmeric, fenugreek and fennel seeds to the pan and fry for a moment, making sure they don't burn. Pour in the mung, rice and veggie mix and give everything a thorough mix before grating in the ginger and seasoning with salt and pepper.
4. Serve with coconut yogurt and coriander.

WILD MUSHROOM RAGU WITH
CREAMY COURGETTI

In this recipe, I use creamy courgetti as a base to pile high with the most comforting plant-based wild mushroom ragu you'll ever taste. It's so rich and hearty, that even the meat lovers in your life will approve. This is mostly down to the addition of a heaped spoonful of miso paste, but the Puy lentils can take a bit of credit too, as they make a great alternative to mince.

Serves 2-3
Prep: 20 minutes
Cook: 20 minutes

RAGU

200 g (7 oz) dried or
250 g/9 oz pack cooked Puy lentils

1 red onion, chopped

2 garlic cloves, minced

avocado or coconut oil, for cooking

200 g (7 oz) chestnut mushrooms,
finely chopped

1 tbsp tomato purée

400 ml (14 fl oz) can of chopped tomatoes

1 tbsp miso paste

100 g (3½ oz) wild mushrooms (chanterelles
and enoki mushrooms are my favourites)

½ tsp cacao powder

a generous pinch of rosemary, finely chopped

200 ml (generous ¾ cup) boiling water

COURGETTI

2 medium courgettes

1 ripe avocado

2 tbsp olive oil

6 fresh basil leaves

2 tbsp nutritional yeast

a handful of leafy greens (cavolo nero,
chard, spinach etc)

salt and black pepper

1. If you're cooking your lentils from dry, pop them on to boil now for 20 minutes. If using a pre-cooked pack (definitely not cheating in my opinion!), skip this step.

2. Place the red onion and garlic in a large pan over a medium heat with a dash of oil. Leave to brown before adding the chestnut mushrooms.

3. Add the cooked puy lentils and stir in the tomato purée. Add the chopped tomatoes and miso paste and season generously. Add the remaining ragu ingredients and leave to cook for 20 minutes.

4. Meanwhile, make your creamy courgetti by spirilising the courgettes (if you don't have a spiriliser, grab a few pre-made packs). Place all the remaining ingredients except the leafy greens in a food processor or blender to make the cream, and blend for a good few minutes until its completely smooth and lump free.

5. Chop the leafy greens and add to the courgetti. Massage in the avocado basil cream using your hands. Once the ragu is cooked, pile it high on top of the creamy courgetti.

BROWN RICE SPAGHETTI WITH SPRING GREENS ● ● ● ●

Greens, glorious greens. My favourite way to pack in those beautiful phytonutrients is to hide them among foods I adore, smothered underneath herby and flavoursome sauces and dressings. You're much more likely to maintain a healthy and well-balanced diet if you just can't get enough of the food on your plate. This springtime favourite is super easy to pull together, packed full of good-for-you ingredients with an underlying happiness that comes only from a big bowl of spaghetti.

Serves 2

Prep: 10 minutes

Cook: 20 minutes

200 g (7 oz) brown rice spaghetti

avocado or extra virgin olive oil, for cooking

1 garlic clove, minced

180 g (6 oz) peas, fresh or frozen

a generous handful of spring greens, chopped

1 ripe avocado, peeled, stoned and sliced

1 large courgette or small pack of courgetti

2 tbsp Kale and Garlic Pesto (see page 185)

5 fresh mint leaves

salt and black pepper

1. Boil the spaghetti in a large saucepan of water for about 12 minutes.
2. Heat a second large saucepan with a touch of oil and add the garlic, peas and spring greens. Cook down for two minutes or so, until the peas are soft. Once the spaghetti is cooked, add it to the pan. Try and spoon it straight from the saucepan so that you get a splash of that lovely starchy water. Give everything a good mix. Keep the pan over a low heat, stirring occasionally.
3. Heat a griddle pan and place the sliced avocado facing down with a touch of salt and pepper and a drizzle of oil. Leave it to cook for at least 5 minutes, so that the surfaces catches and grill marks appear.
4. Spiralise the courgette and add the courgetti, pesto and mint to the pan with the spaghetti, giving everything a mix. Leave to cook for a few more minutes before plating up with the grilled avocado on top.

Opt for wholesome brown rice spaghetti as it's free from gluten and gives you a sustainable source of energy throughout the rest of the day. Just make sure that brown rice flour is the sole ingredient.

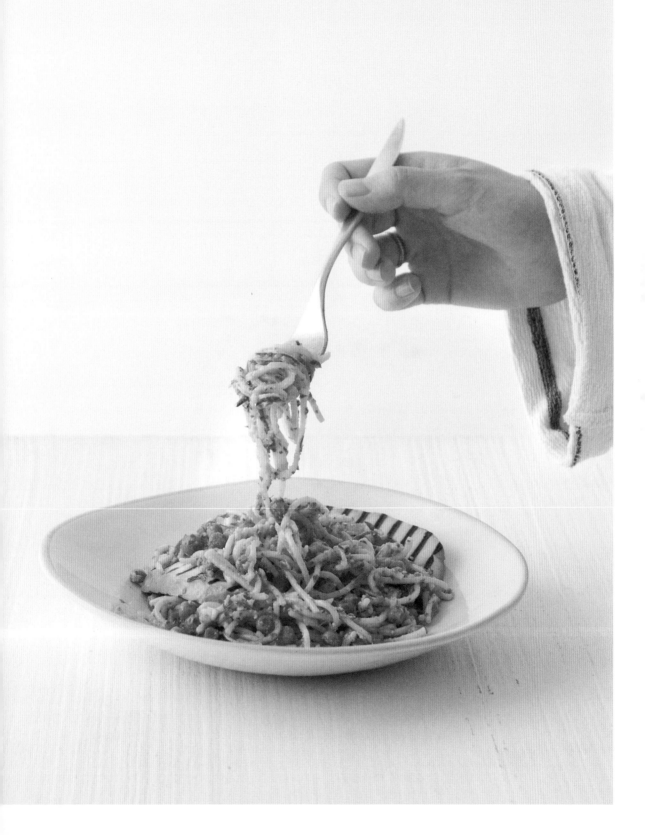

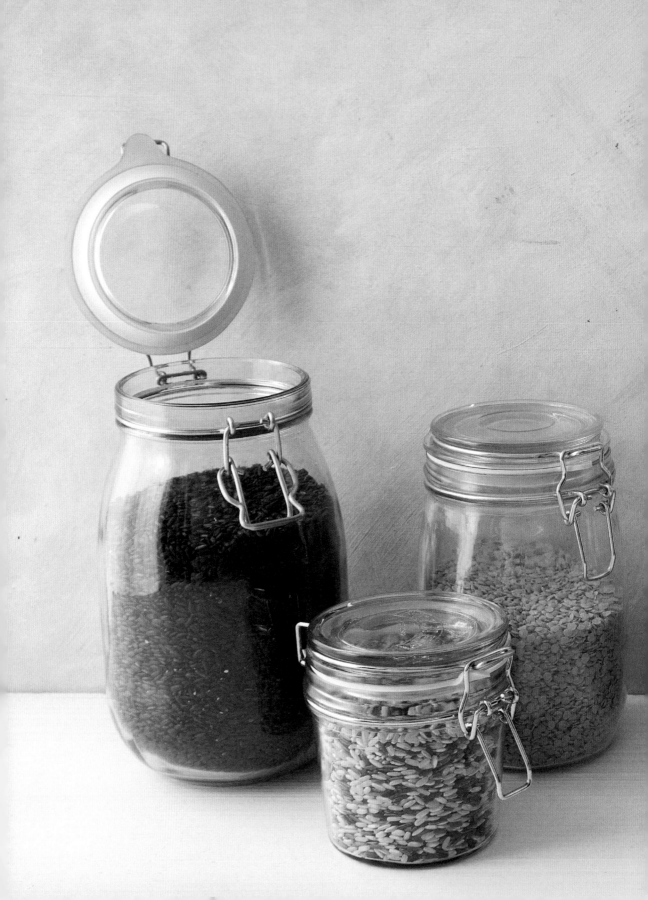

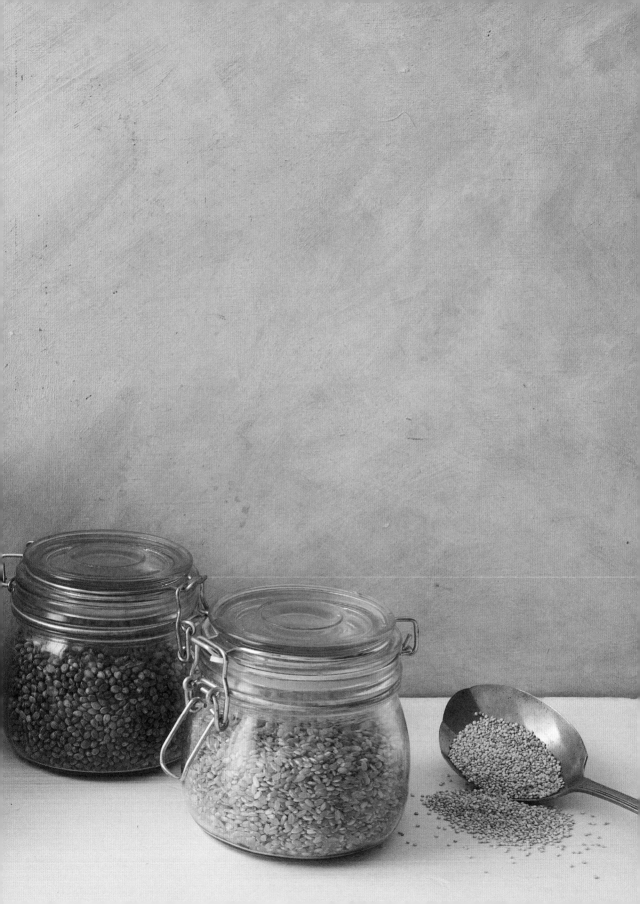

JARRED SALADS

Among the busyness of everyday life, it's easy to become a little bit robotic with our on-the-go meals. However, I don't think anything you eat should be a last resort or purely for convenience. Every meal should excite you and nourish you sufficiently to take on the rest of the day.

Jarred salads are a fabulous option for a grab-and-go lunch, and will give everyone at work major food envy each time they open the fridge. You can eat them cold too, making them a foolproof way to get in a healthy, nutrient-packed lunch.

COLOURFUL PEANUT NOODLE JAR

Makes 1 small jar

Prep: 30 minutes

75 g (2 ¾ oz) buckwheat soba noodles

1 carrot

¼ of a large cucumber

1 raw beetroot, peeled

1 tbsp peanut butter

1 tsp coconut aminios (or tamari)

1 tbsp coconut milk

a small thumb-sized piece of ginger

½ ripe avocado

¼ of a small lime

1 tsp dried chilli flakes (or 1 freshly sliced chilli)

a fistful of flaked toasted coconut

a fistful of fresh coriander, chopped

1. Place the soba noodles in a bowl of lukewarm water to soften for 20 minutes. In the meantime, spiralise the carrot and cucumber, then grate the beetroot. If you don't own a spiraliser, you can simply grate all the ingredients instead. Layer the veggies in the bottom of a small lidded jar.
2. Make a dressing by combining the peanut butter, coconut aminos, coconut milk and a grating of ginger in a small bowl before setting aside.
3. Once the noodles are cooked, drain them and thoroughly rinse in cold water before placing into the jar, and pouring over the peanut dressing.
4. Chop the avocado into small chunks or slices and place it on top of the noodles, giving it a squeeze of lime juice to ensure it stays fresh. Throw the remaining ingredients into the top of the jar, seal, and store in the fridge until ready to eat.

If you're sensitive to soy, then coconut aminos can be a great alternative to soy source or tamari. It has the same rich taste that can add a lovely depth of flavour to your dishes, from satay style sauces to soups.

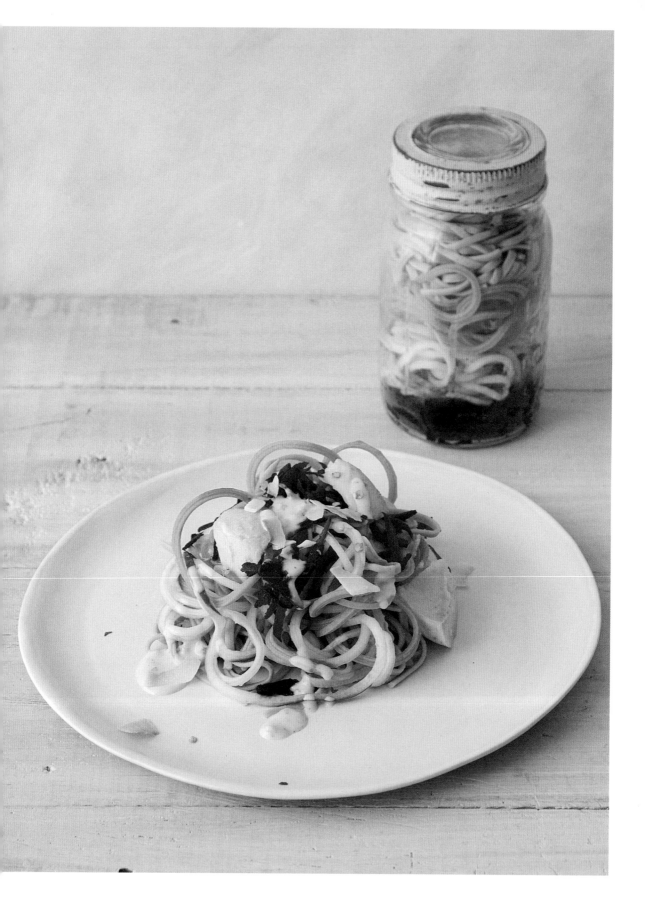

MUSHROOM, SWEET POTATO
AND ALMOND BUTTER JAR

● ● ● ●

Makes 1 small jar
Prep: 15 minutes
Cook: 40 minutes

1 medium sweet potato

avocado oil, for cooking

50 g (1¾ oz) quinoa, rinsed
    thoroughly

50 g (1¾ oz) Puy lentils (or
    use precooked ones)

1 tsp Brazil Nut Pesto (see
    page 182)

1 large portobello
mushroom (about
    100 g/3½ oz), sliced

1 tsp coconut aminos or
    tamari

1 tbsp almond butter

a fistful of toasted
pumpkin seeds

1. Preheat the oven to 200°C/400°F/gas mark 6.
2. Slice the sweet potato into thin coins, place on a baking tray with a drizzle of avocado oil and bake for about 20 minutes.
3. Meanwhile, boil the quinoa in a saucepan with 250ml (1 cup) water over a medium heat. If you're using dry Puy lentils, throw them in as well. If they are pre-cooked, put them a separate pan to heat through for a few minutes before setting aside. Leave the quinoa to cook for 15 minutes, until it has soaked up all the water. Once cooked, stir in the pesto and spoon the quinoa into the bottom of your jar, along with Puy lentils if precooked.
4. Gently fry the mushroom in a pan with a touch of avocado oil and garlic. Add a splash of coconut aminos and leave the mushroom to soak up all the flavour for 5 minutes or so.
5. Layer the baked sweet potato on top of the quinoa, then the mushroom. Finish with a dollop of almond butter and pumpkin seeds. Seal the jar and store in the fridge until ready to eat.

Superfood Kale

Kale is one of the most hormone-healthy ingredients you can add to your diet. It's high in folic acid and packed full of incredible minerals, from calcium to magnesium. Just be sure to avoid eating it raw, as it's harsh on digestion and contains goitrogens, a no-go for PCOS sufferers and those with thyroid issues.

Cooking with Mushrooms

Mushrooms cooked well can completely transform a dish, so give them some love. A generous drizzle of oil should go into the hot pan first, before throwing in mushrooms that have been wiped clean with a paper towel, along with minced garlic and herbs. Give them enough room to cook and don't overcrowd the pan or bother them too much. You want the flat surface to catch a nice colour before plating up.

Anti-inflammatory Foods and Hormones

A body in balance goes hand in hand with a diet high in anti-inflammatory foods. Opting for real, whole foods – particularly powerful inflammation-fighting ingredients, such as turmeric, ginger, olive oil and even good-quality dark chocolate – gives you a head start in tackling unruly hormones head on. Recipes crammed full of anti-inflammatory superheroes are especially useful to have on hand during your menstrual phase.

BEETROOT AND PORTOBELLO MUSHROOM STEW WITH CELERIAC MASH

● ● ● ●

My favourite type of vegetarian food shouts about vegetables from the rooftops, celebrating every sweet carrot, fragrant fennel bulb and peppery rocket leaf, and this stew is the perfect example of giving vegetables that little bit of love with a long, slow cook.

Puy lentils and hefty portobello mushrooms are the perfect way to bulk up any dish, as well as packing an extra plant-based protein punch. Pile on top of creamy celeriac mash, for a lovely light alternative to mashed potato. Celeriac is lower in carbohydrates and contains high amounts of B6, an essential vitamin for balanced hormones and healthy progesterone production.

Serves 4
Prep: 15 minutes
Cook: 1 hour

STEW

1 red onion, sliced
avocado or coconut oil, for cooking
400 g (14 oz) raw beetroot, peeled and roughly chopped
150 g (5 ½ oz) baby carrots, topped
2 garlic cloves, minced
1 vegetable stock cube
700 ml (3 cups) boiling water
1 tbsp tomato purée
150 ml (2/3 cup) red wine
1 ½ tbsp brown miso paste
3 large portobello mushrooms, sliced
250 g (9 oz) pre-cooked Puy lentils (from a pack or boiled for 15 minutes)
2 sage leaves
a generous pinch of thyme sprigs
salt and black pepper

CELERIAC MASH

1 garlic clove, minced
2 medium-sized celeriac, peeled and cut into small chunks
a drizzle of olive oil
salt and black pepper

1. Preheat the oven to 180°C/350°F/ gas mark 4.
2. Put the red onion in a large ovenproof pan or casserole dish over a medium heat with a drizzle of oil. Fry until browned, then add the chopped beetroot, carrots and garlic. Dissolve the stock cube in a jug with the boiling water.
3. Stir the tomato purée into the vegetables and add the wine. Leave to reduce for about 5 minutes before adding half the veggie stock and the miso paste. Cook for 30 minutes, stirring occasionally.
4. Add the portobello mushrooms to the pan or dish with the pre-cooked Puy lentils. Pour in the remaining veggie stock and add the sage leaves and thyme. Transfer to the oven and bake for 20 minutes.
5. Once the stew is in the oven, make the celeriac mash. Heat a large saucepan, add a glug of oil along with the garlic and chopped celeriac. Give it a minute or so before completely covering with boiling water and leave to simmer for 20 minutes, until soft. Drain the water and blend in a food processor or blender with some salt and pepper to taste. Serve with the stew piled on top.

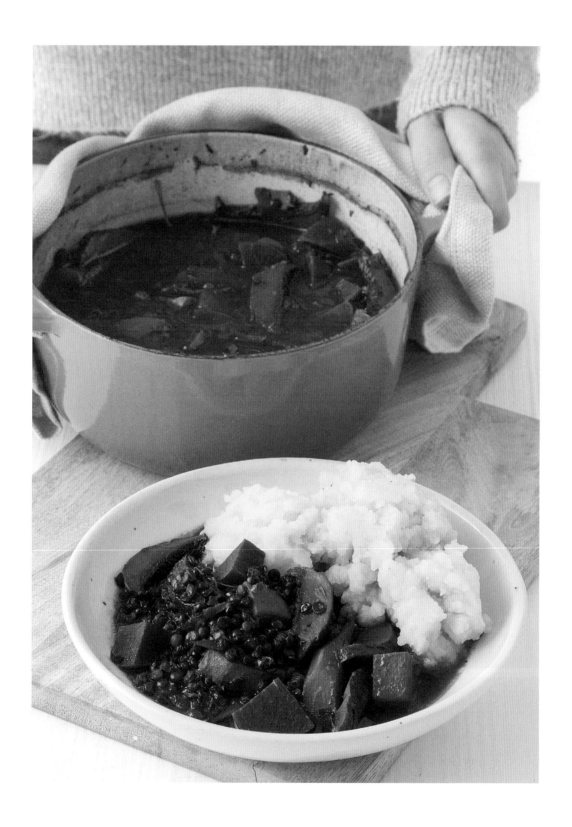

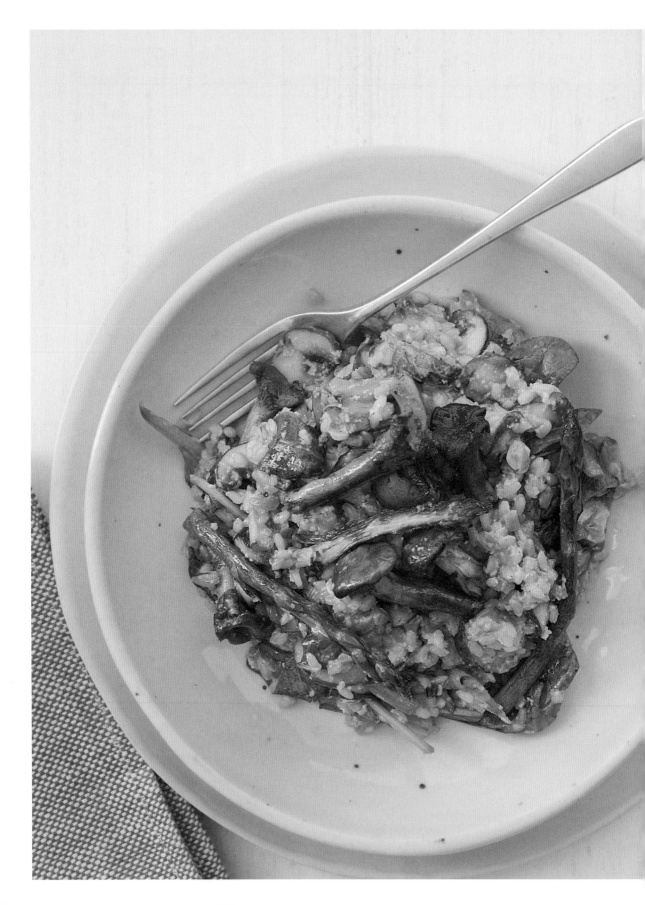

CHANTERELLE MUSHROOM AND ASPARAGUS RISOTTO WITH CASHEW CREAM

● ● ● ●

I try to eat seasonally where possible, for a number of reasons, the main one being taste. Take asparagus, for example. During asparagus season, you'll see thick green spears wrapped tightly in colourful rubber bands everywhere you look. When cooked right, they are juicy yet maintain a slight crunch at the same time.

Slice into fine ribbons and toss into a creamy jumble of short-grain brown rice, meaty golden chanterelles, seasonal greens and you have yourself a wholesome, healthy risotto. Packed full of vegetables and with the addition of cashew cream, it's high-fat and anti-inflammatory due to an abundance of greens.

Serves 2

Prep: 15 minutes, plus soaking overnight

Cook: 55–60 minutes

200 g (1 cup) short-grain brown rice (ideally soaked overnight in cold water)

600 ml (2 ½ cups) boiling water

1 vegetable stock cube or 1 tbsp of veggie stock powder

50 g (½ cup) cashews (soaked for at least an hour)

4 tbsp nutritional yeast

avocado or coconut oil, for cooking

1 onion, finely chopped

1 large garlic clove, minced

125 g (4 ½ oz) chestnut mushrooms, sliced

a generous pinch of thyme sprigs

100 g (3 ½ oz) asparagus, sliced in half lengthways

100 g (3 ½ oz) chanterelle mushrooms (or any other wild mushroom), washed and dried

2 handfuls of seasonal leafy greens

salt and black pepper

crushed roasted hazelnuts and a drizzle of extra virgin olive oil, to serve

1. Rinse the soaked rice thoroughly and place it in a saucepan with the boiling water and the stock cube. Bring back to the boil over a medium heat and then leave to simmer for 40 minutes, until all the water has been absorbed.

2. Place the soaked cashews in a food processor or blender along with the nutritional yeast and about 100 ml (scant ½ cup) water. Blend until completely smooth and a lump-free cream forms.

3. Just before the rice has finished cooking, heat a second pan and add a dash of oil. Throw in the onion and garlic. Give them a few minutes to cook down, letting the onion brown slightly. Add the chestnut mushrooms and thyme.

4. Give the mushrooms a moment to cook before adding the asparagus ribbons – they should catch slightly and start to brown. Add the chanterelle mushrooms.

5. Throw in the cooked brown rice, cashew cream and seasonal leafy greens. Season generously with salt and pepper to taste. Cook for another 5 minutes or so and feel free to add a touch more water if needed. Serve with the crushed roasted hazelnuts dropped on top and a drizzle of olive oil.

LENTIL SHEPHERD'S PIE WITH CREAMY CASHEW AND SWEET POTATO MASH

● ● ● ●

This is my kind of comfort food. Food that quite literally hugs you warm, making the madness of your everyday life mute, if only for a brief moment. It's the type of food that not only makes your body feel good, but makes your soul overflow. Come the arrival of the colder seasons, I make a giant plant-based shepherd's pie at least once a week and pick away at the remains for the days that follow. From the skin saviour that is delicious sweet potato, to the protein-packed mushroom and Puy lentil filling, it really is healthy home cooking at its best.

Serves 4-5

Prep: 15 minutes, plus 4 hours soaking

Cook: 10-15 minutes

550 g (1 ¼ lb) raw sweet potatoes (about 2 large), peeled and chopped

1 red onion, chopped

avocado or coconut oil, for cooking

2 garlic cloves, minced

250 g (9 oz) chestnut mushrooms, finely minced

250 g (9 oz) pack pre-cooked Puy lentils

1 large carrot, finely chopped

100 g (3 ½ oz) peas, fresh or frozen

400 ml (14 oz) can chopped tomatoes

1 tbsp tomato purée

1 tbsp dark miso paste

a pinch of dried thyme

a generous handful or two of seasonal leafy greens

75 g (½ cup) cashews, soaked for at least 4 hours (in cold water)

5 tbsp nutritional yeast

100 ml (scant ½ cup) almond milk

salt and black pepper

1. Preheat the oven to 200°C/400°F/gas mark 6.
2. Place the sweet potato in a steamer basket and steam for about 10–15 minutes or so, until soft. Meanwhile, place the onion in a large pan with a dash of oil over a medium heat and fry until browned.
3. Add the minced garlic, mushrooms, pre-cooked Puy lentils, carrot, peas, chopped tomatoes, tomato purée, miso, thyme and leafy greens and season generously. Leave to simmer for 20 minutes or so.
4. Once the sweet potatoes are soft, place them in a food processor or blender and blitz until fluffy.
5. Remove about three-quarters of the sweet potato mash and set aside. Drain the soaked cashews and then add to the remaining mash along with the nutritional yeast, almond milk and some seasoning. Blend again until completely smooth.
6. Once the filling is cooked, transfer to a large ovenproof dish and top with the plain sweet potato mash and smooth down. Top with the creamy mash and smooth down. Bake for 40 minutes until golden and crispy on top.

Nut allergy? Swap the cashews for sunflower seeds if you need to avoid nuts. They'll need a longer soak, overnight is optimal, but work just as well.

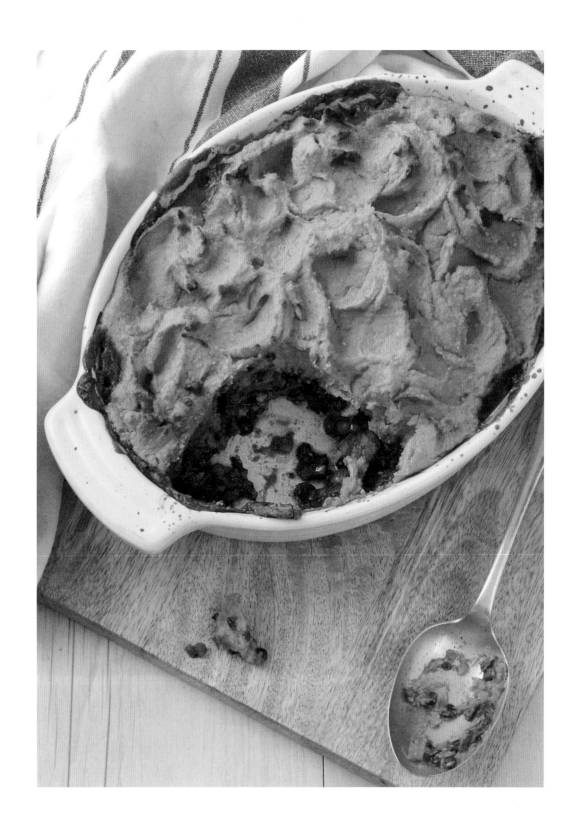

SPELT FLATBREAD WITH TURMERIC ROASTED CAULIFLOWER AND BLACK QUINOA

● ● ● ●

Spelt is a truly marvellous ancient grain, with a delicate and nutty flavour. Packed with protein it provides a prolonged release of energy, instead of instantly spiking blood sugar. There are two different ways to cook this beautiful cruciferous vegetable for this recipe: baking cauliflower leaves it ever-so-slightly crispy on the edges, yet with a lovely roasted flavour on the inside. On the other hand, boiling lightly – until it's soft enough to stick your fork through – before chargrilling, leaves it lighter with a slightly charred flavour. Both methods make this sometimes tricky vegetable shine.

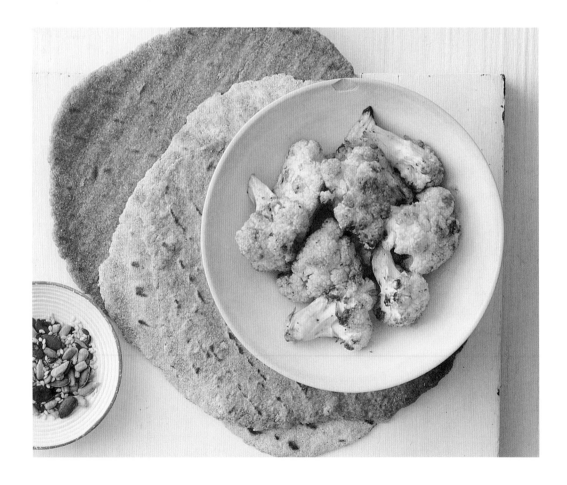

Serves 2

Prep: 20 minutes, plus soaking overnight

Cook: 30 minutes

400 g (14 oz) cauliflower, chopped into florets

a generous drizzle of extra virgin olive oil or avocado oil

1 tsp ground turmeric

½ tsp ground cumin

80 g (3 oz) black quinoa (ideally soaked overnight in cold water)

a few generous handfuls of cavolo nero or any other leafy green

1 tbsp Brazil Nut Pesto (see page 182)

a generous dollop of dairy-free coconut yogurt

25 g (1 oz) pumpkin seeds, toasted

25 g (1 oz) sunflower seeds, toasted

2 tbsp of fresh coriander, chopped, to serve

1 tbsp pre-made pink pickled onions, to serve (optional)

salt and black pepper

FLATBREADS

200 g (2 cups) sprouted spelt flour

2 tbsp dairy-free coconut yogurt

1 tbsp extra virgin olive oil

a pinch of salt

1. Preheat the oven to 200°C/400°F/gas mark 6. Line a baking tray with baking parchment. Spread out the chopped cauliflower on the tray and drizzle with oil. Sprinkle with the turmeric and cumin and season generously with salt and pepper. Using your hands, rub the seasoning all over the cauliflower and then bake for 20 minutes until golden and crispy.

2. Place the quinoa in a saucepan with double the amount of boiling water and leave to simmer away for 15–20 minutes.

3. Make the flatbreads by combining all the ingredients with 4 tbsp cold water in a large bowl and kneading with your hands until the dough holds together well. Add a touch more water or flour to reach the desired consistency if needed. Roll out into two individual flatbreads on a floured surface, then rest on an open flame on the stove top to cook, constantly turning, until each surface catches slightly.

4. Once the quinoa is cooked and absorbed all the water, add the leafy greens and stir in the pesto. Assemble your flatbreads by smothering them with the coconut yogurt then topping with quinoa and leafy greens and turmeric cauliflower. Finish with a sprinkling of toasted seeds, fresh coriander and a few slices of pink pickled onion on each.

If you would prefer, you can boil the cauliflower in a saucepan for about 5 minutes until you can easily stick a fork through it. Drain, brush it with the oil, turmeric and cumin and place it on a griddle pan over medium/high heat to chargrill for at least 10 minutes.

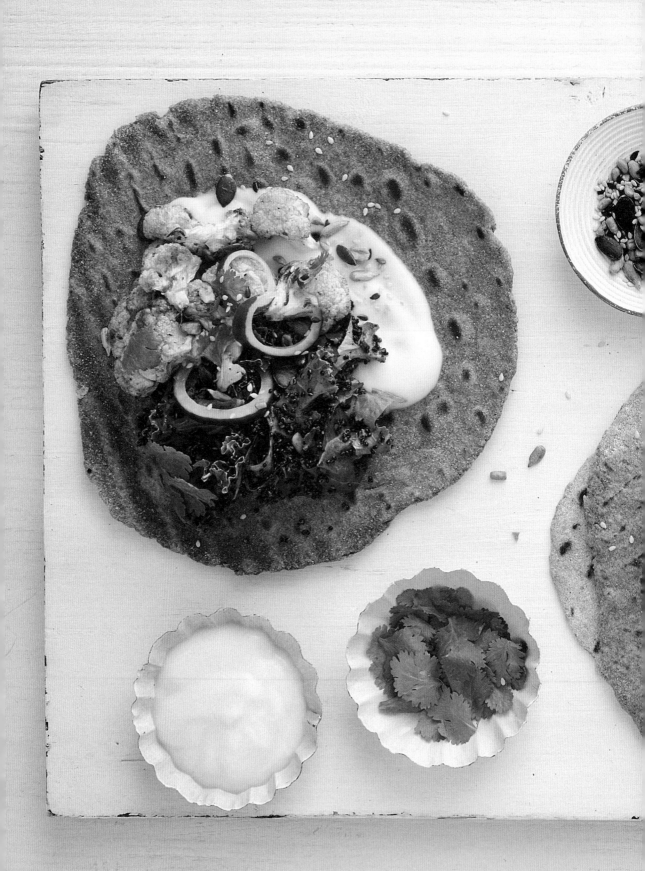

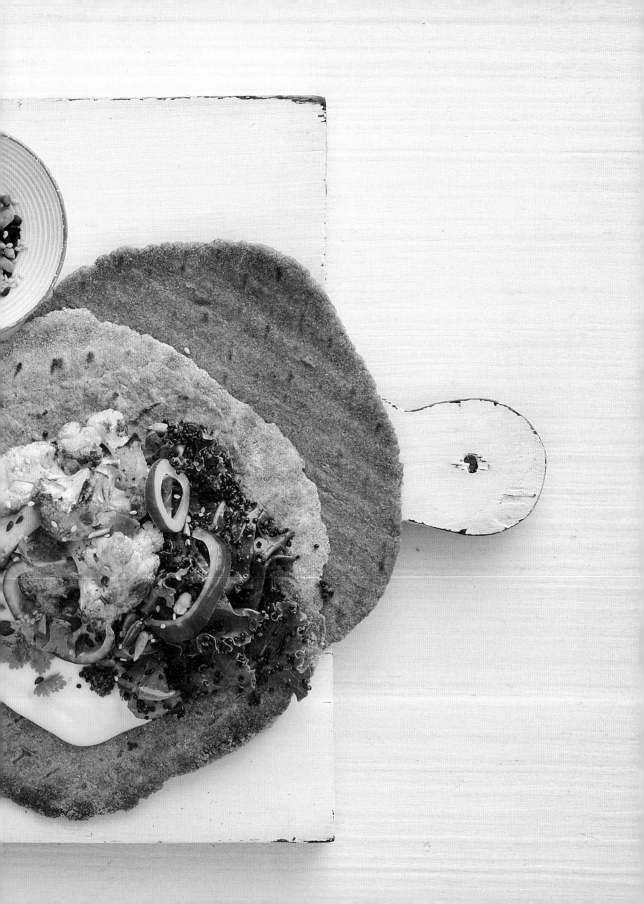

BEETROOT AND CARROT BURGERS
WITH SATAY SLAW

● ● ● ●

As much as I love big comforting autumnal bowls of food, as soon as the weather starts to change, I am instantly drawn to lighter dishes filled with fresh vegetables. These burgers are just that: they're wonderfully vibrant, succulent and a real crowd pleaser, ready to be flung onto the barbecue on a hot summer's day.

The satay slaw accompanying this recipe is the perfect pairing. Cabbage is amazing for the liver, aiding in the detoxification of used oestrogen and peanut butter is rich in healthy fat, so dig in if you're ever feeling slightly off-balance.

Serves 4-6

Prep: 15 minutes plus 4 hours soaking

Cook: about 1 hour

170 g (½ cup) short-grain brown rice (soaked, ideally for at least 4 hours)

400 ml (14 oz) can chickpeas, drained and rinsed

1 tbsp tahini

4 tbsp extra virgin olive oil

2 garlic cloves, smashed

60 g (½ cup) toasted pumpkin seeds

300 g (10½ oz) raw beetroot, grated

3 carrots, grated

a small thumb-sized piece of ginger, grated

salt and black pepper

SATAY SLAW

2 tbsp coconut cream

2 tbsp peanut butter, crunchy or smooth

1 tbsp coconut aminos or tamari

2 large carrots, grated

¼ head of cabbage, red or white, finely sliced

a 3cm piece of ginger

1. Boil the brown rice in a saucepan of water for 30 minutes.
2. Preheat the oven to 180°C/350°F/gas mark 4. Line a baking tray with baking parchment.
3. Start making the bugers by placing the rinsed and drained chickpeas in a food processor or blender with the tahini, olive oil, garlic and toasted pumpkin seeds. Blitz until the chickpeas are smashed and the mix becomes creamy.
4. Put the grated beetroot in a large pan over a medium heat and cook down slightly; this will only take a couple of minutes. Add the cooked beetroot to the food processor, along with the grated carrots, ginger and the cooked brown rice, just for a moment until everything is combined yet still a little chunky.
5. Take large handfuls of the mix and mould into patties with your hands. Place on lined baking tray and bake for 30 minutes. Feel free to throw onto the barbecue once cooked – they'll only need an extra 5 minutes or so to get those lovely grill marks.
6. While the burgers are cooking, whip up the satay slaw. Mix together the coconut cream, peanut butter and coconut aminos and generously mix into the grated carrots and cabbage in a large bowl. Grate over a touch of fresh ginger and serve the slaw either on top of the burgers or as a side.

Use the pulp from the Sunshine Juice on page 65 in place of the grated beetroot and carrot for this recipe. Add in a splash of the juice as well for optimal flavour.

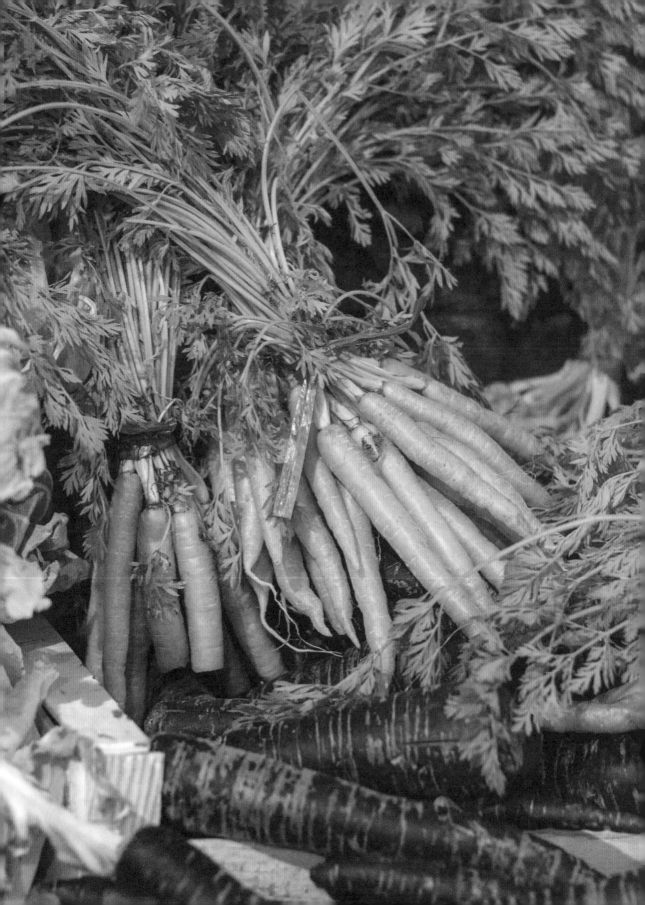

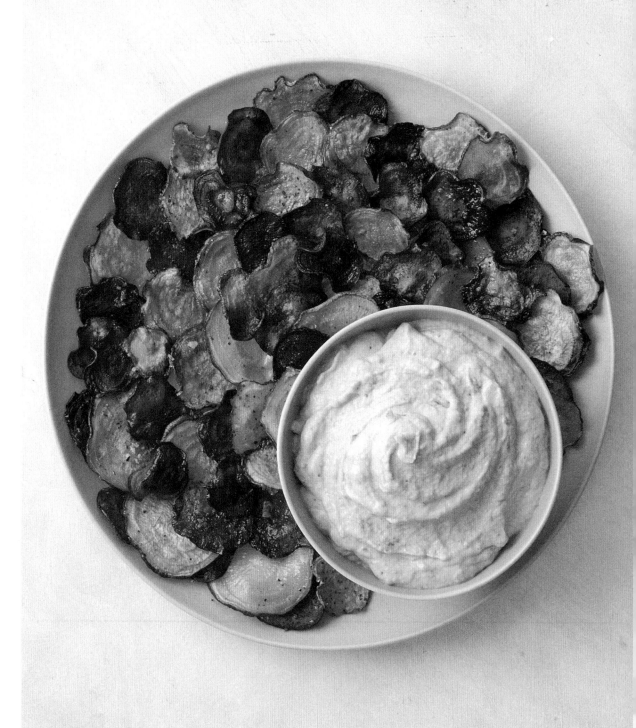

RAINBOW BEETROOT CRISPS
WITH BABA GANOUSH

● ● ● ●

You can never have just one vegetable crisp. They're one of the most moreish snacks going, and you can bet that at any gathering, be it Christmas drinks or a summer barbecue, you'll find me beside the bowl, scoffing away. They're actually surprisingly easy to make yourself, and paired with intensely smokey, homemade baba ganoush, make for the ultimate healthy crowd pleaser. The smell of burning aubergines on an open flame as they blister away is up there as one of the most satisfying food smells, and is almost as delightful as eating the finished dip.

Serves 4 as a side
Prep: 5 minutes
Cook: 15-20 minutes

BEETROOT CRISPS

3-4 large raw
beetroots (golden,
candy and / or red)

a pinch of flaked sea salt

a crack of black pepper

a few sprigs of
fresh rosemary

BABA GANOUSH

2 aubergines

1 tbsp tahini

a squeeze of lemon juice

a lug of extra
virgin olive oil

salt and black pepper

1. Preheat the oven to 200°C/400°F/gas mark 6. Line 2 baking trays with baking parchment.

2. Slice the top and base off the beets and scrub until clean, making sure you dry them well. Thinly slice either by hand or using a mandolin – I've found the thickness of a 10p coin to be optimal.

3. Place on the lined trays so the beets are spread evenly. Season generously with a crack of black pepper, sea salt and a few sprigs of rosemary. Bake for 15–20 minutes until crisp.

4. Meanwhile, place each aubergine on an open flame on the stove top and allow to completely blister as you keep turning them to ensure an even burn. This should take around about 5 minutes and the aubergines should go completely soft.

5. Once cooled, carefully strip each aubergine of its skin and place the soft flesh into a food processor or blender along with the rest of the baba ganoush ingredients. Blitz until smooth, then serve alongside the crisps.

COCONUT AND CASSAVA
FLOUR TORTILLA CHIPS

● ● ● ●

Every party and intimate gathering needs a big bowl of tortilla chips planted in the centre of the table for people to nibble away at. Instead of grabbing the first packet of oversized tortilla chips you find on the supermarket shelf, why not try making your own? I love baking with coconut flour as it has the sweetest flavour, and is gluten, nut and grain-free, making it an all-round people pleaser. This also goes for cassava flour, which is easily digestible, exactly what you want from an ingredient you'll be shovelling into your mouth by the handful.

Serves 4–6 as a side
Prep: 15 minutes
Cook: 25 minutes

65 g (½ cup) coconut flour

130 g (1 cup) cassava flour

½ tsp baking powder

a drizzle of melted coconut oil (about 1 tbsp)

a pinch of sea salt

1. Preheat the oven to 180°C/350°F/gas mark 4.
2. Combine the flours and other ingredients in a large mixing bowl with 375 ml (1½ cups) water. Knead together to form a ball of dough.
3. Place a sheet of baking parchment on a flat surface and place the ball of dough in the centre. Place another sheet of parchment on top and using a rolling pin, gently flatten the mix. Ideally, you want to get the dough as thin as possible without it breaking.
4. Place the sheet with the rolled dough onto a baking tray and slice into triangles. Give each one a brushing of coconut oil and a pinch of sea salt before baking for about 20–25 minutes until slightly golden. Halfway through the bake, I like to give each one a flip to ensure an even bake.

CHARGRILLED MISO BABY GEM LETTUCE

● ● ● ●

Lettuce, often a bit of a sad vegetable, can be completely transformed by simply brushing with oil and chargrilling. It's a complete game changer, worthy of a place on any table. I adore the richness of miso and it's the perfect way to give any veggie side dish that little bit of extra love. Serve at big family barbecues in place of burger buns, alongside gloriously fresh pasta bowls or even to be nibbled on as a fancy snack. The way the lettuce softens slightly and grabs hold of the salty miso is worth going the extra mile.

Serves 4

Prep: 5 minutes

Cook: 5 minutes

1 tbsp dark or light miso paste

2 tsp maple or brown rice syrup

2 tsp coconut aminos or tamari

4 baby gem lettuce heads, sliced in half lengthways

a fistful of black or white sesame seeds, fresh coriander and dried chilli flakes, to finish

1. Preheat a griddle pan or a barbecue.
2. Mix together all the liquid ingredients in a small bowl. Dip each side of the lettuce into the bowl, then place cut-side down onto the hot griddle pan or on the barbecue. Grill for 5 minutes before serving sprinkled with a fistful of sesame seeds, chopped coriander leaves and a pinch of chilli flakes.

JEWELLED WILD SAFFRON RICE

● ● ● ●

Sometimes we simply cook up a batch of rice and plop it down on the side of our plates without giving it a second thought. It's typically an understated accompaniment to the main part of your meal. How about instead, we make it the star of the show? This tumble of wild rice with sweet-flaked almonds, chewy dried apricots and wonderfully warming spices will not just look magical sitting on your table, it will taste glorious too. Pair it with stews, curries or simply pick away at it on its own.

Serves 4

Prep: 15 minutes, plus 4 hours soaking

Cook: 30 minutes

200 g (7 oz) wild rice, (soaked, ideally for at least 4 hours in cold water)

1 tbsp coconut butter

a generous pinch of saffron threads

40 g (1½ oz) flaked almonds

40 g (1½ oz) roasted pistachios, finely chopped

10 g (⅓ oz) parsley, finely chopped

10 g (⅓ oz) coriander, finely chopped

40 g (1½ oz) pumpkin seeds, toasted

100 g (3½ oz) pomegranate seeds

10 dried apricots, finely chopped

a light pinch of ground cinnamon (preferably Ceylon)

1. Start by placing the rice on to boil for about 30 minutes. About half way through the rice cooking, place the coconut butter in a small saucepan with a dash of boiling water and the saffron threads and melt over a gentle heat for five minutes . Thoroughly mix until a paste is formed and set aside.

2. Once cooked, drain and rinse the rice with cold water. Place in a large pan over a low heat and fold in the saffron-infused coconut butter to completely coat the rice.

3. Transfer to a large bowl and toss through the chopped nuts and herbs, before topping with the pomegranate seeds, dried apricots and a pinch of cinnamon.

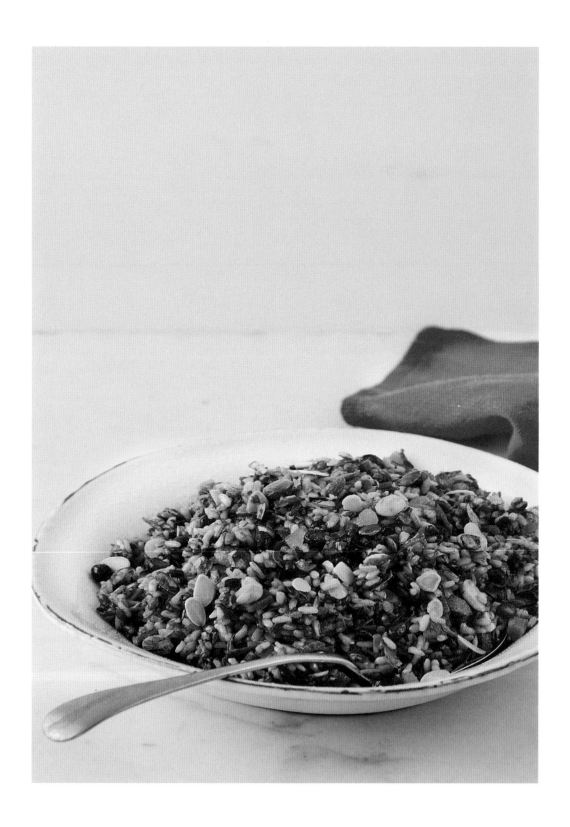

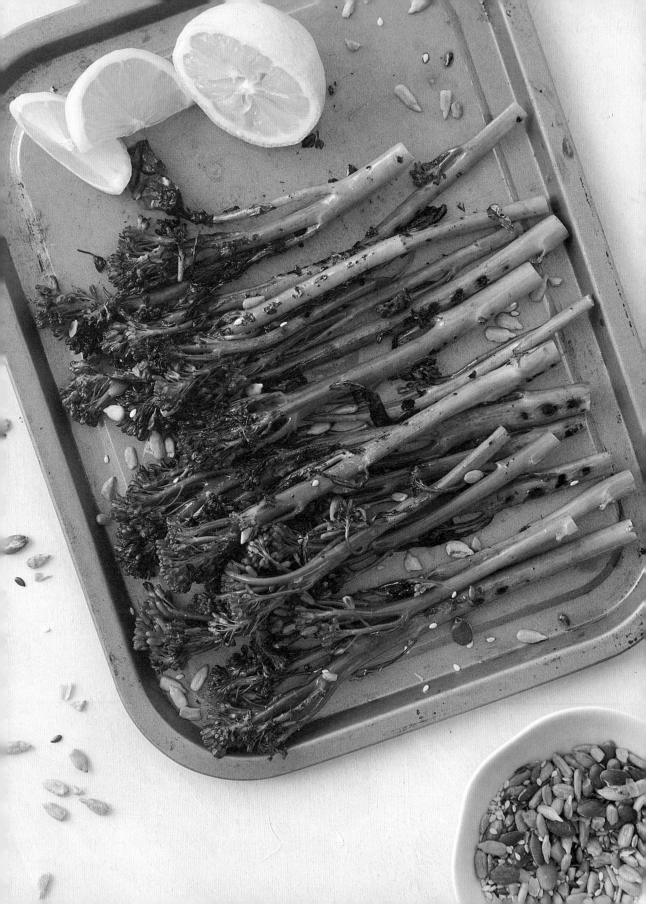

ZESTY CHARGRILLED BROCCOLI

● ● ● ●

Cruciferous veg, like broccoli, should be a staple in any hormone-healthy diet, due to their oestrogen-balancing properties, blood sugar stabilising and nutrient dense profile. While steamed broccoli isn't one of the most appetising side dishes, there are many other ways you can make this fabulous green taste incredible. By chargrilling in a drizzle of avocado oil, you're getting a dose of healthy fats, while a grating of lemon zest transforms the flavour.

Serves 4

Prep: 5 minutes

Cook: 5 minutes

a drizzle of avocado oil

300 g (10 ½ oz) Tenderstem broccoli

1 lemon

salt and black pepper

a fistful of sunflower and pumpkin seeds, to serve

1. Heat a griddle pan and add a drizzle of avocado oil. Place the tenderstem broccoli in the pan so that the grill marks will run horizontal. Cook for 5 minutes, flipping halfway through, before grating over the zest from the lemon and seasoning with salt and pepper.
2. Add a quick squeeze of lemon juice, if desired, and serve with the seeds sprinkled over the top.

Snacks & Sweets

GOLDEN COCONUT MILK

● ● ● ●

Golden milk, also known as the popular turmeric latte, is a wonderfully comforting alternative to your morning coffee. It's a hormone health godsend, from the intensely anti-inflammatory properties of both turmeric and ginger (two essential ingredients when hormonal breakouts and painful PMS come knocking), to the gorgeously fatty coconut butter and milk. Coconut butter not only helps to keep you satiated, but is also highly antibacterial and another skin saviour. I like to add a dash of ashwagandha powder into my golden milk for it's calming and soothing effects on the nervous system, giving the body that extra helping hand when combatting stress.

Serves 1

Prep: 5 minutes

Cook: 5 minutes

250 ml (1 cup)
coconut milk

½ tsp ground turmeric

½ tsp ground cinnamon
(preferably Ceylon),
plus extra for dusting

¼ tsp ground ginger
or freshly grated

a crack of black pepper

a scraping of seeds
from a vanilla pod (or ·
teaspoon vanilla powder)

½ tbsp coconut butter

½ tsp ashwagandha
powder

1. Place all the ingredients, except the coconut butter and ashwagandha, into a saucepan over a low to medium heat and whisk everything together. Leave to simmer for 5 minutes.
2. Lastly, whisk in the coconut butter and ashwagandha and leave for a further minute. Pour into your mug and finish with a dusting of cinnamon on the top.

MUSHROOM HOT CHOCOLATE
WITH COCONUT CREAM

Mushrooms? In hot chocolate? Let me explain. The benefits of medicinal mushrooms (see Tip below) are endless, from boosting the immune system to nurturing the adrenals, through to helping protect the body against symptoms of stress. It just makes sense to be adding them into your hormone-healthy diet. Pairing mushrooms with glorious and antioxidant rich cacao will have you reaching for this recipe time and time again. It's thick and creamy, making for the most perfect treat to come home to after a long day, sipped while cuddled up on the sofa. Top with whipped vanilla coconut cream, because you deserve it.

Serves 2

Prep: 5 minutes, plus 10 minutes soaking

Cook: 5 minutes

500 ml (2 cups) plant-based milk (see pages 178–179)

2 medjool dates, stoned (soaked for at least 10 minutes in warm water)

2 ½ tbsp raw cacao powder

1 tbsp coconut or almond butter

½ tsp chaga mushroom powder

½ tsp reishi mushroom powder

400 ml (14 oz) can full-fat coconut milk (thick cream removed from top)

a scraping of seeds from a vanilla pod

½ tsp maple syrup (optional)

1. Place all the ingredients, with the exception of the coconut cream, vanilla seeds and maple syrup, in a food processor or blender and blend together. Pour the liquid into a saucepan over a medium heat and leave to simmer for about 5 minutes or so.

2. Meanwhile, place the coconut cream in a bowl. Add a scraping of vanilla seeds (done by simply slicing the pod and scraping out roughly a 2.5 cm (1 in) worth of bean) and a touch of maple syrup, if desired. Whisk together until smooth.

3. Pour the hot chocolate into two mugs, topping each with a generous dollop of the whipped coconut cream.

Chaga and reishi mushrooms are a wonderful adaptogenic addition to a creamy hot chocolate, made either with homemade nut milk or full-fat coconut milk. You can buy them in powder form from your local health-food store, or better yet, opt for a multi-mushroom mix including a number of different varieties.

ICED VANILLA CASHEW CHAI

● ● ● ●

Considering what kind of concoction you can make from that gallon of homemade cashew milk you've just pressed and is now sitting in the fridge? Give this iced vanilla chai a go, slurp away on the sweet yet warming combination of spices and revel in the pride of making your own milk from scratch. While chai lattes are typically reserved for the colder seasons, an iced chai finished with an extra dusting of cinnamon can make the perfect cooler for sunnier times when your taste buds just aren't in favour of another fruity cocktail.

Serves 1

**Prep: 5 minutes, plus
1 hour chilling**

Cook: 5 minutes

3 cardamom pods,
seeds removed

2 cloves

½ tsp ground cinnamon
(preferably Ceylon)

a crack of black pepper

250 ml (1 cup) Cashew
Milk (see page 179)

a small piece of ginger

a scraping of seeds
from a vanilla pod

1 tsp coconut or
almond butter

ice cubes, to serve

1. In a small saucepan, gently toast the seeds from the cardamom pods, the cloves, cinnamon and black pepper over a low heat before slowly adding the cashew milk. Grate in the ginger and add the vanilla seeds before leaving to simmer for 5 minutes. Just before the 5 minutes is up, add the coconut butter and whisk.

2. Leave the mix to completely cool before pouring into a jug and transferring to the fridge to chill for an hour. Add a few ice cubes to a glass and pour your cashew chai over. You can also enjoy warm if preferred.

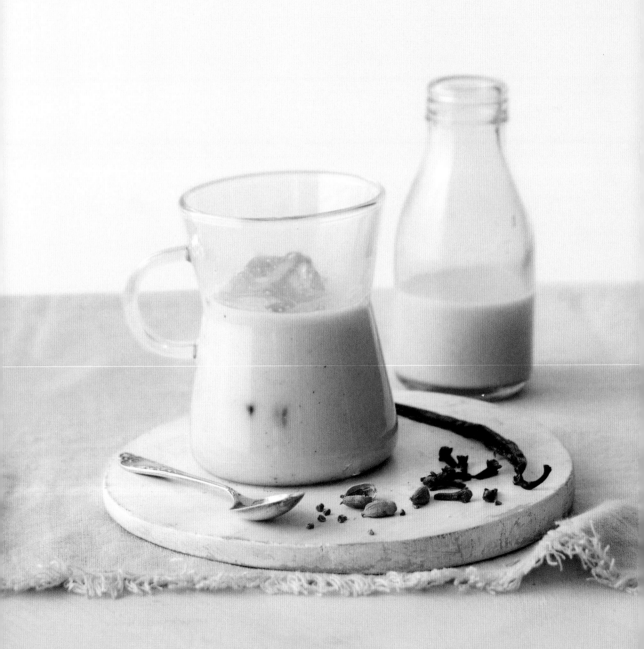

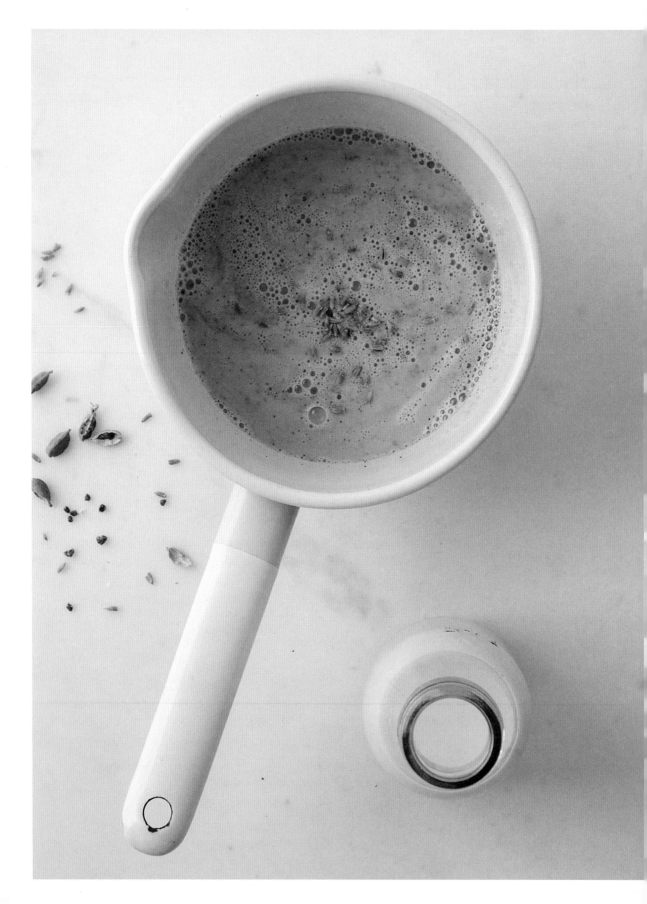

SOOTHING LAVENDER BEDTIME MILK

● ● ● ●

I believe we don't put enough emphasis on the quality of sleep: deep sleep is essential for reaching peak performance, both in physical and mental health. When you're young, you're given a mug of warm milk to help you drift off into a sleepy slumber, so let's take that concept and give it a bit of a spruce. Pour a lug of homemade plant-based milk into a pan and watch as it bubbles away with soothing spices and vibrant pods of lavender.

Serves 1

Prep: 5 minutes

Cook: 5 minutes

250 ml (1 cup) plant-based milk (see pages 178-179)

2 cardamom pods, seeds removed

½ tsp ashwagandha powder

½ tsp ground cinnamon (preferably Ceylon)

5 individual lavender pods or 1 drop of essential oil

a scraping of seeds from a vanilla pod

½ tsp maple syrup or honey (optional)

1. Pour the milk into a small saucepan over a low–medium heat. Grind the cardamom pods and add to the milk along with the remaining ingredients. Leave to simmer away for 5 minutes or so. Feel free to fish out the lavender pods just before you're ready to drink, or leave them in.

MATCHA UPGRADES

I consider myself rather lucky that I despise the taste of coffee. Coffee is the thing that we typically won't negotiate on, and for most of us, that's fine. However, if your adrenals are in overdrive and the rest of your endocrine system, from your thyroid to your liver, is feeling a little rundown, I highly recommend rethinking your alliance. Matcha is a great alternative if you're looking to cut down a bit. It gives you that lovely perky feeling, without the jitters. It has also been said to create a little bubble of calm among the storm of hectic life, giving you the best of both worlds – productivity without becoming a maniac.

CINNAMON-SPICED MATCHA

Serves 1
Prep: 5 minutes
Cook: 5 minutes
½ tsp matcha green tea powder
250 ml (1 cup) plant-based milk (see pages 178-179)
½ tsp ground cinnamon (preferably Ceylon)
1 tsp almond butter

BEETROOT AND ROSE MATCHA

Serves 1
Prep: 5 minutes
Cook: 5 minutes
½ tsp matcha green tea powder
250 ml (1 cup) plant-based milk (see pages 178-179)
½ tsp beetroot powder or 1 tsp beetroot juice
½ tsp rosewater
edible rose petals, to top

COCONUT MATCHA

Serves 1
Prep: 5 minutes
Cook: 5 minutes
½ tsp matcha green tea powder
250 ml (1 cup) coconut milk
1 tsp coconut butter

For all matcha recipes:
1. Add the matcha powder to a mug with a dash of hot (not boiling) water and mix to create a paste.
2. Heat up the milk and the rest of your ingredients in a saucepan over a low-medium heat for about 5 minutes. Pour the milk into the cup with the matcha and whisk gently before drinking.

CHOCOLATE HAZELNUT MILK

● ● ● ●

I truly believe that there is not a single flavour combination out there more joyous than hazelnut and chocolate. It's a combination that brings back fond memories of sneakily taking large spoonfuls of Nutella straight from the jar when no one was looking. Nutella lovers rejoice, as this recipe is quite literally liquid gold. Best served iced or warmed up on the stove for a couple of minutes for the ultimate hot chocolate.

Serves 2

Prep: 5 minutes, plus

30 minutes soaking

Cook: 5 minutes (optional)

500 ml (2 cups)
Hazelnut Milk
(see page 178)

1 medjool date, stoned
(soaked for at least
30 minutes in warm water)

1 tbsp Hazelnut Butter
(see page 180)

1½ tbsp cacao powder

1. Place all the ingredients in a food processor or blender and blend until completely smooth. Serve chilled or pour into a saucepan and heat gently for 5 minutes and serve hot.

NOURISH BALLS

Nourish balls are conveniently shaped and sized, allowing you to pack for a long run, eat on the walk home from the gym or simply as a mid-afternoon boost. The natural sweetness from the dates provides a lovely surge of energy when you need it most, without the drastic blood sugar spike that many shop-brought energy drinks or bars will give. They're also a great source of fibre, which is key for optimal digestion.

I'll pack each ball full of healthy fats, from coconut butter to almond butter, as well using nuts as a key base ingredient. This is where the nourish part comes into play. These types of monounsaturated fats nourish cells and help maintain healthy hormone function. Take them to the next level by adding your favourite adaptogens and superfoods, such as chaga mushroom powder for immune function, or maca powder known for both its energising and hormone balancing properties.

Now, onto the fun bit. From peanut butter to matcha, there are endless ways of jazzing up nourish balls. In my opinion, the best flavours include chocolate and cardamom, lemon and poppy seeds and sea salted caramel. The addition of cardamom into a chocolate base is a welcome twist and gives each individual ball a fragrant boost that lingers well after the snack has disappeared. The lemon and poppy seed is a slightly lighter, fresher taste, and don't even get me started on sea salted caramel! What's not to love? These little bursts of goodness are practically mini desserts in the form of a healthy snack.

CHOCOLATE AND CARDAMOM NOURISH BALLS

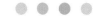

Makes 8-12 balls
Prep: 10 minutes

6 cardamom pods, seeds removed

150 g (1 cup) almonds, skin on

10 medjool dates, stoned

2 tbsp coconut or almond butter or coconut oil

2 tbsp raw cacao powder

2 tbsp maca powder

1. Grind the cardamom seeds in a pestle and mortar. This can be a fiddly job, but from a flavour perspective, it's really worth it. Set aside once ground.
2. Place the almonds in a food processor or blender, blitzing them until broken. Add the remaining ingredients, including the ground cardamom seeds. Blend until a sticky dough forms and holds together well.
3. Roll the dough into 8-12 golf ball-sized rounds. Keep in the fridge until ready to eat. They will keep for up to a week.

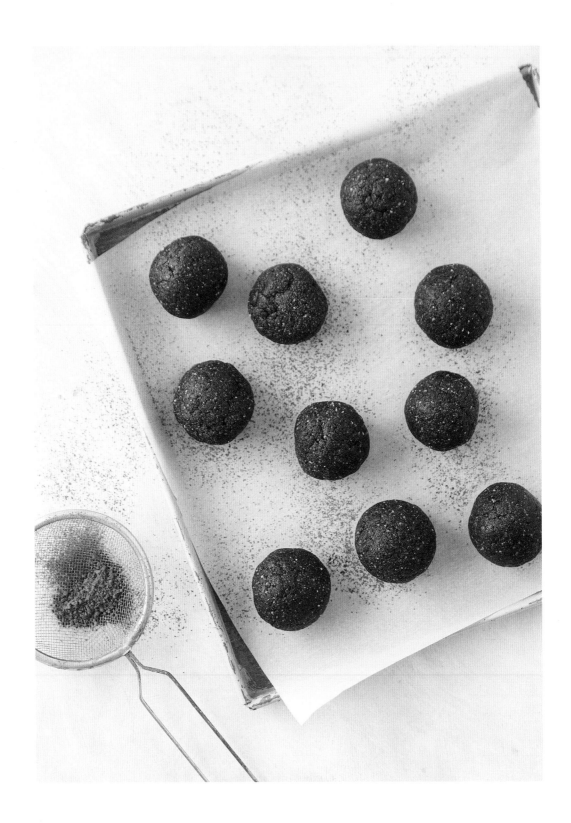

LEMON AND BLACK SESAME SEED
NOURISH BALLS

Makes 8–12 balls

Prep: 10 minutes

150 g (1 cup) cashew nuts

12 medjool dates, stoned

2 tbsp almond butter

1 tbsp lemon juice

grated zest of 1 lemon

2 tbsp maca powder

80 g (3 oz) oats

2 tbsp black sesame seeds

1. Place the cashews in a food processor or blender and blitz until broken. Add the dates, almond butter, lemon zest and juice, and maca. Blend until a sticky dough forms and holds together well.
2. At the final moment, add the oats and black sesame seeds. Blend again until everything is combined.
3. Roll the dough into 8–12 golf ball-sized rounds. Keep in the fridge until ready to eat. They will keep for up to a week.

SALTED MACA CARAMEL NOURISH BALLS

Makes 8–12 balls

Prep: 10 minutes

150 g (1 cup) pecans

10 medjool dates, stoned

1 tbsp coconut butter or coconut oil

2 tbsp maca powder

a pinch of sea salt

1. Place the pecans in a food processor or blender and blitz until broken. Add the remaining ingredients and blend until a sticky dough forms and holds together well.
2. Roll the dough into 8–12 golf ball-sized rounds. Keep in the fridge until ready to eat. They will keep for up to a week.

COCONUT BUTTER CUPS

● ● ● ●

I like my snacks full of fat to keep me full and focused throughout the day, but most importantly, to rival the taste of anything I could buy in a shop. When you munch on foods you actually want to eat, as opposed to simply eating to fuel the latter part of your day, eating well becomes a lot less complex. Take these coconut butter cups, for example. The sheer pleasure that comes from eating a wonderfully creamy layer of pure coconut butter, sandwiched between rich dark chocolate, is unbeatable. They're nourishing and full of those good for you nutrients that'll ensure stabilised blood sugar when you need it most.

Makes 12 cups

Prep: 5 minutes, plus 15 minutes setting

Cook: 5 minutes

200 g (7 oz) good-quality dark chocolate (85% cocoa solids)

12 tbsp coconut butter, softened

sea salt flakes

1. Line a 12-hole cupcake tin with cuocake cases.
2. Melt the dark chocolate in a small bowl over a pan of simmering water. Spoon a tablespoon of the melted chocolate into each cupcake case, then transfer to the fridge for 15 minutes or so to harden.
3. Once the first layer has set, spoon over a tablespoon of softened coconut butter into each before covering with the remaining melted chocolate and a pinch of sea salt to finish. Store in the fridge for 1 hour to set.

Mix things up by swapping coconut butter for peanut butter, almond butter or even homemade hazelnut butter (see page 180).

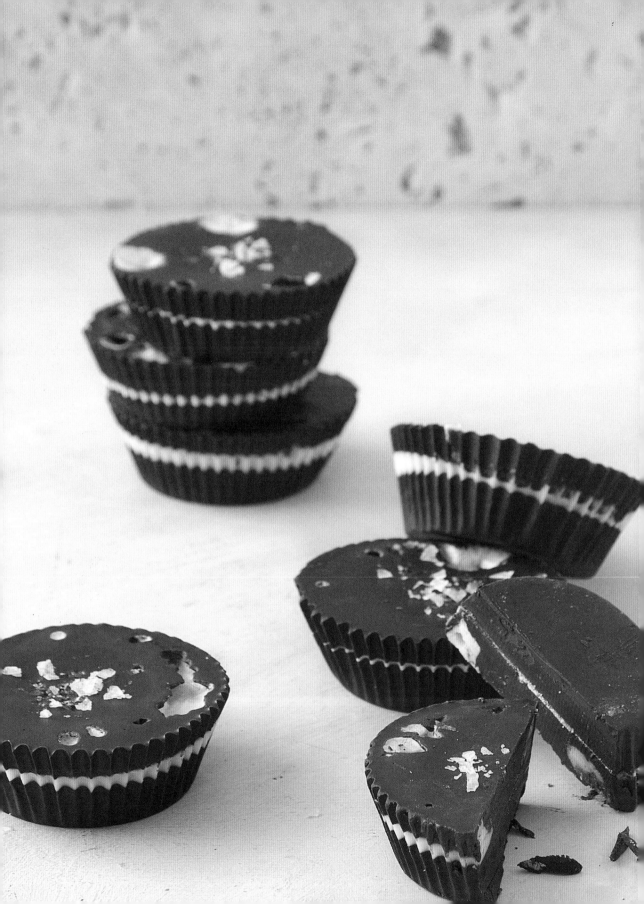

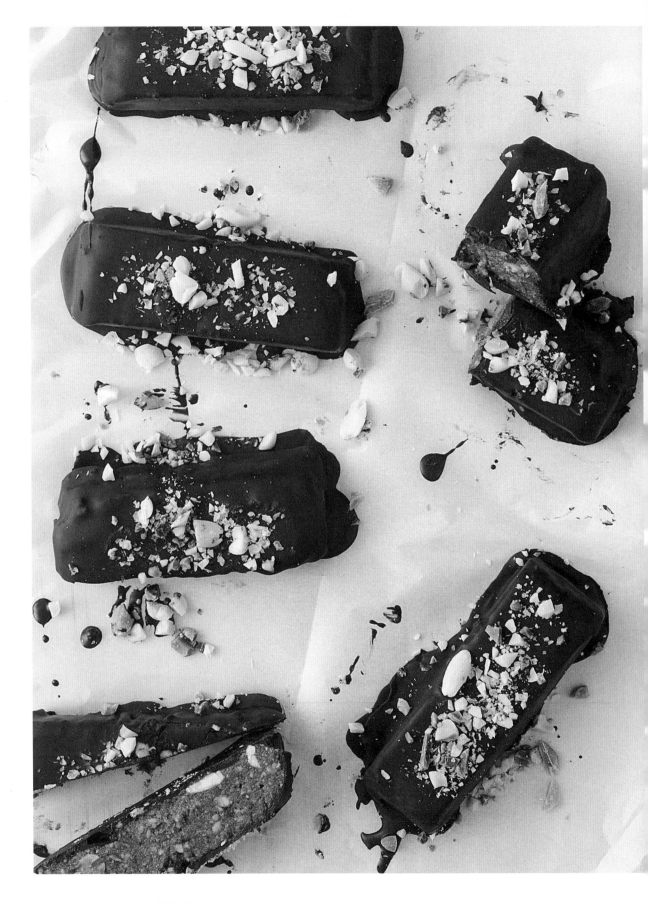

CHOCOLATE PEANUT BARS

● ● ● ●

I wish I could tell you that I've got my peanut butter addiction under control, but in all honesty, life is too short to be weighing out your PB, so eat up! Luckily, peanut butter can be a fabulous hormone-healthy ingredient. It's healthy fat packed and high in plant-based protein. Add dollops to smoothies, spread it thickly on warm homemade bread and blend generous amounts into chocolate coated raw treats. I love this recipe because each individual bar is ridiculously gooey, with whole roasted peanuts adding the most amazing crunch.

Makes: 6 bars or 12 bite-sized squares

Prep: 10 minutes, plus 1 hour soaking and 2½ hours chilling

12 medjool dates, stoned (soaked for 1 hour in warm water)

4 generous tbsp peanut butter, crunchy or smooth

2 tbsp maca powder (optional)

150 g (5½ oz) roasted peanuts

150 g (5½ oz) good-quality 85% solids dark chocolate

sea salt and a handful of crushed peanuts, to top

1. Place the dates, peanut butter and maca powder into a food processor or blender and blend until completely smooth, gradually adding in a touch of the date soaking water as needed to help blend. It should be thick with no lumps.
2. Add half the roasted peanuts, pulsing for a couple of seconds until slightly broken up, before folding in the rest with a spoon.
3. Line a loaf tin with baking parchment and pour in the mix. Smooth it down using the back of a spoon, making sure the mix is level and spread equally. Transfer to the freezer for at least 2 hours to set.
4. Once set, remove from the tin and slice into roughly 5 cm (2 in) thick bars, or smaller bite-sized squares if preferred.
5. Melt the dark chocolate in a bowl over a saucepan of simmering water. Completely submerge the frozen bars in the melted chocolate – I find using two forks helps. Place on a board lined with fresh baking parchment, sprinkle over a few extra crushed peanuts and sea salt before placing the fridge to further set for 30 minutes.

In warmer months, keep the bars in the freezer for ice cream bars.

SALTED ALMOND AND
BUCKWHEAT ROCKY ROADS

● ● ● ●

There's a lot to be said for raw(ish) desserts, made from real, nourishing ingredients. When you're craving a chocolate bar, the last thing you want is a kale smoothie. So instead, grab something even more delicious that also happens to make you feel wonderful.

If you're looking for the perfect pairing of salty and sweet, this recipe is for you, with its combination of naturally sweet medjool dates and scatter of sea salt flakes on the surface. These moreish bars are full of fibre and packed with healthy fats. From whole roasted almonds to almond and cacao butter, they're superb for your hormone health, skin and, of course, your happiness.

Makes 8–12 squares

Prep: 15 minutes, plus overnight soaking and 1 hour chilling

200 g (1¼ cups) almonds, skins on

100 g (1 cup) activated buckwheat (soaked overnight and left to dry)

10 medjool dates, stoned (soaked for 10 minutes in warm water)

5 tbsp smooth almond butter

80 g (3 oz) cacao butter or 4 tbsp coconut oil

4 tbsp raw cacao powder

a pinch of sea salt

1. Preheat the oven to 200°C/400°F/gas mark 6. Roast the almonds for about 10 minutes. They should smell heavenly by this point. Set aside to cool completely.
2. Toast the soaked, dried buckwheat gently in a dry pan. Set aside to cool completely.
3. Place the dates in a bowl of warm water and leave to soften for at least 10 minutes. Once soft and gooey, pop the dates into a food processor or blender along with 4 tablespoons of the water they were soaking in and the almond butter. Blend until completely smooth. This may take a few minutes.
4. Melt the cacao butter or coconut oil in a bowl set over a pan of simmering water. Once liquid, pour into the food processor along with the cacao powder. Blend until a thick, fudgy consistency forms.
5. Add half the roasted almonds to the food processor and blitz for a moment until slightly crushed. Fold in the rest of the almonds, the toasted buckwheat and sea salt to ensure lots of whole, crunchy pieces remain.
6. Pour the mix into a loaf tin that has been lined with baking parchment, smoothing it down with the back of a spoon until evenly spread. Ideally, you want the rocky roads to be lovely and thick. Transfer to the freezer for at least 1 hour to set. Once hard, cut into generous squares. Keep in the fridge until ready to eat.

RAW ALMOND BUTTER AND CHOCOLATE SLICES

● ● ● ●

Nut butters are a staple in my kitchen. Almond butter, the best of the bunch in my opinion, is indulgently creamy with a slightly salty taste, and, unlike peanut, doesn't dominate other flavours. Therefore, it makes the perfect filling in this recipe, sandwiched between a wonderfully gooey base and a solid, homemade chocolate top.

Better still, almond butter is crammed full of monounsaturated fats, great for keeping blood sugar levels stable and, therefore, creating harmony among the rest of your hormones. It also contains vitamin E – the ultimate glow-giving nutrient – and is high in magnesium and iron.

Makes 8–10 slices

Prep: 10 minutes, plus 2½ hours chilling

BASE

220 g (1½ cups) almonds, skin on

medjool dates, stoned

2 tbsp maca powder

1½ tbsp coconut butter or coconut oil

20 g (¼ cup) desiccated coconut

a pinch of sea salt

ALMOND BUTTER LAYER

100g smooth almond butter

CHOCOLATE LAYER

80 g (3 oz) cacao butter

2 tbsp raw cacao powder

2 tbsp smooth almond butter

(or use one 100g bar of good-quality 85% cocoa solids dark chocolate)

1. Start by blitzing the almonds in a food processor or blender until crumbly and no large pieces remain. Add the remaining base ingredients and blend until a sticky dough forms.
2. Line a tin (I've found a loaf tin works well here) with baking parchment and press the dough firmly into the base, ensuring it's even and tightly packed. Spread the almond butter onto the base – you can place the tin onto the scales and weigh out the amount then and there. Smooth with the back of a spoon and place in the freezer to completely set for 2 hours.
3. Just before the 2 hours are up, melt all the chocolate layer ingredients in a bowl resting over a simmering saucepan of water, whisking to ensure everything is combined and lump free.
4. Drizzle the chocolate over the almond butter layer until completely covered. Set in the fridge for a further 30 minutes. Once solid, slice into roughly 2.5 cm (1 in) thick slices and keep in the fridge until ready to eat.

BEETROOT BROWNIES WITH
CHOCOLATE HAZELNUT ICING

● ● ● ●

Licking the remains after slaving away over a decadent brownie batch is, in my option, almost as satisfying as eating the finished product. Plant-based brownie recipes have been popping up left, right and centre for the last couple of years, and for good reason. From sweet potato to black bean bases, adding extra fibre into your baked goods is key for optimal digestion and takes away the need for refined sugar. Instead, I've sweetened these beetroot brownies with gooey medjool dates and packed in the antioxidants with rich cacao and of course, beetroot, for glowing skin and balanced hormones.

Makes 10–12 brownies

Prep: 30 minutes

Cook: 25 minutes

10 medjool dates, stoned

200 ml (1 cup) warm water

300 g (10½ oz)
raw beetroot

80 g (3 oz) rolled oats
(if gluten sensitive, use
gluten-free oats)

80 g (3 oz) ground
almonds

6 tbsp raw cacao powder

6 tbsp coconut oil, melted

50 g (1¾ oz) dark
chocolate (at least
70% cocoa solids),
broken into chunks

CHOCOLATE
HAZELNUT ICING

80 g (½ cup) roasted
hazelnuts (roughly
10 minutes in the oven,
until the skins spit
and fall away easily)

4 tbsp coconut
butter or oil

2 tbsp raw cacao powder

1 tsp maple syrup
(optional)

1. Submerge the dates in the warm water. Leave to soak as you start the first part of the recipe. Preheat the oven to 180°C/350°F/gas mark 4.

2. Peel and chop the beets into small chunks before steaming until completely soft. This should take about 20 minutes in a steamer basket.

3. Place the rolled oats in a food processor or blender and blend until a fine flour forms. Place the oat flour in a large mixing bowl and mix with the ground almonds and cacao.

4. Once the beetroots are soft, place them in a food processor or blender with the soaked dates, the date water and the melted coconut oil. Blend until completely smooth and thick. There should be no lumps remaining.

5. Add the beetroot and date mix to the dry ingredients and mix until everything is combined, folding in the dark chocolate chunks to finish.

6. Pour the mix into a 20 cm (8 in) square baking tray that has been lined with baking parchment and spread evenly. Bake for 25 minutes.

7. To make the icing, simply combine the roasted hazelnuts, coconut butter, cacao powder and maple syrup (if using) in a food processor or blender, blend until completely smooth. Spread on the brownies once completely cooled and slice into pieces, as little or large as you like.

RAW-ISH PEANUT BUTTER AND CHOCOLATE CHEESECAKE

These are a real treat, and a nod to the time in my life when I discovered that I could in fact make cheesecake somewhat healthy. Our fridge saw every flavour under the sun, from chocolate orange to raspberry vanilla, all as creamy and delightful as the next. The winning combination, in my opinion, is peanut butter and chocolate. The base is crunchy, while the filling is wonderfully creamy. It's sweet, without being overtly sickly, and can be make into one large round cheesecake or several individual square towers.

Makes 8–10 individual cheesecakes, or one large cheesecake

Prep: 10 minutes, plus overnight soaking and 1 hour chilling

BASE

140 g (5 oz) peanuts (roasted, for better flavour), plus a few extra crushed peanuts, to decorate

8 medjool dates, stoned

1 tbsp cacao powder

2 tbsp cacao nibs

1 tbsp coconut butter or oil

FILLING

300 g (2 cups) cashews (soaked overnight)

3 medjool dates, stoned (soaked for at least 30 minutes in warm water)

4 tbsp of the date soaking water

80 g (3 oz) coconut oil, melted

140 g (5 oz) peanut butter, smooth or crunchy

2 tbsp maple syrup

2 tbsp cacao powder

a couple of squares of dark chocolate, to decorate

1. Make the base by combining all the base ingredients in a food processor or blender and blitzing for a couple of moments. You want it sticky enough to hold together, but still containing some larger chunks of peanuts.
2. Press the base into the bottom of a tin – I like to use either a standard loaf tin for square cheesecakes or a small round cake tin for slices. Ensure it's tightly packed and level.
3. To make the creamy filling, add all the filling ingredients, with the exception of the cacao, into the processor, blending until completely smooth. This may take a good few minutes. Once smooth, transfer half the mix to a bowl, add the cacao to the remaining half and blend until combined.
4. Layer the plain peanut butter half onto the base, smoothing down to ensure it is even before smoothing over the cacao layer. Place in the freezer for an hour to set, before transferring to the fridge. Top with a few extra crushed peanuts and a drizzle of dark chocolate.

NUT-FREE SALTED CHOCOLATE TART

It's been a mission of mine to create a ridiculously delicious dessert free from nuts, for my best friend Bea who has a serious nut allergy. Unless you have a life-threatening allergy, you probably are unaware of how many plant-based treats contain nuts. But worry not, pumpkin, sunflower and sesame seeds have your back. Better yet, seeds are lovely and high in those wonderful monounsaturated fats, helping with healthy hormone production and function.

Serves 12–16 people

Prep: 10 minutes, plus 1½ hours chilling

BASE

40 g (1½ oz) pumpkin seeds

40 g (1½ oz) sunflower seeds

7 medjool dates, stoned

3 tbsp coconut oil

40 g (½ cup) rolled oats

2 tbsp raw cacao

FILLING

5 medjool dates, stoned

2 tbsp coconut oil

4 tbsp raw cacao

45 g (1½ oz) creamed coconut (hard) or 4 tbsp cream off the top of a can of coconut milk

1 tbsp maple syrup (optional)

sea salt flakes, to top

1. Toast all the seeds lightly in a dry frying pan until they start to pop, this should only take a few minutes. Soak the dates for the filling in a bowl of warm water for 10 minutes. Set both aside.

2. Blend all the base ingredients together in a food processor or blender, with the exception of the seeds, until crumbly. Add the seeds at the last moment and blitz for a minute until combined. You ideally still want the seeds whole and crunchy, however this is completely up to you. Blend for longer if you like smaller chunks.

3. Firmly press the seedy, chocolate mix into a 20 cm (8 in) round tart tin that has been base-lined with baking paper. Create a slightly thicker crust that climbs a little way up the side of the tin, making sure that the dough is tightly packed down. Transfer to the freezer to set for at least 30 minutes.

4. Drain the dates and keep the soaking water. Just before the base has set, place all the filling ingredients in the food processor or blender along with 4 tablespoons of the date soaking water and blend on a high speed for a good few minutes until completely smooth and free from any lumps. The mix should be thick and creamy.

5. Spread the filling in the set tart case, ensuring it is level. Sprinkle a touch of sea salt on top and transfer to the fridge to set for a further hour. Feel free to get fancy with your toppings such as drizzled melted chocolate, fresh fruit or edible flowers – have fun with it.

This recipe is the perfect luteal phase recipe, for the days where you're feeling sluggish and chocolate seems to be the only thing on your mind. Both the pumpkin seeds and rich cacao powder are high in magnesium, great for combatting fatigue.

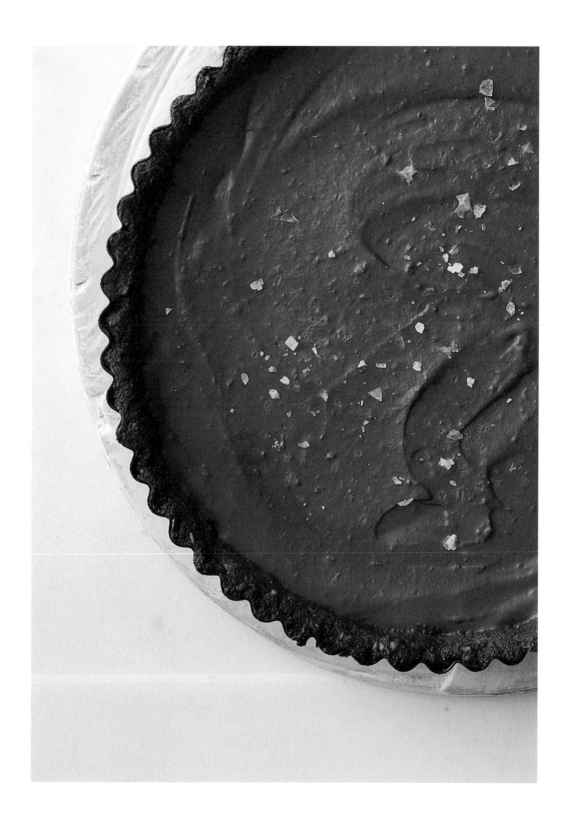

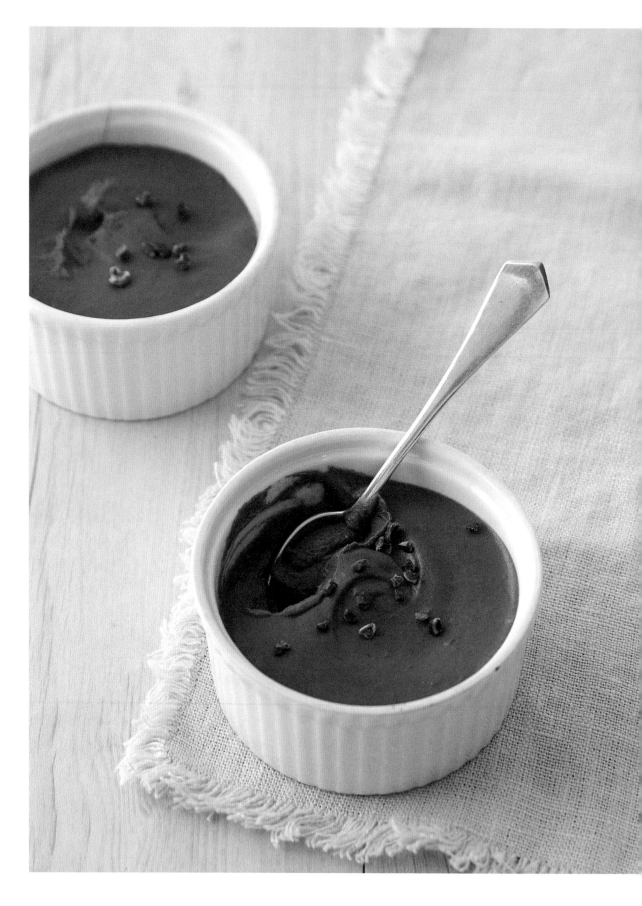

SWEET POTATO CHOCOLATE MOUSSE

I might be biased, but there is a high chance this going to be the most moreish, drool-worthy dessert you will ever make. With its thick and creamy consistency, it will take every ounce of your willpower to resist scraping it from the blender and straight into your mouth. It's also not overbearingly sweet, allowing you to eat as much as your heart desires.

This particular chocolate mousse recipe is packed full of nourishing, nurturing ingredients such as skin savours sweet potato (vitamin E) and raw cacao (antioxidants), plus rich coconut cream that promotes healthy hormone production.

Serves 2-4

Prep: 10 minutes, plus
1 hour soaking and
30 minutes chilling

Cook: 20 minutes

1 sweet potato (about
315 g/11 oz), peeled and
chopped into small chunks

4 tbsp cacao powder

3 medjool dates, stoned
(soaked for at least
1 hour in warm water)

400 ml (14 oz) can
full-fat coconut milk
(all the cream on top
plus up to 4 tbsp of
the coconut milk)

1. Steam the sweet potato until completely soft, in a steaming basket, this should take around 20 minutes or so.
2. Once soft, place the sweet potato in a food processor or blender along with the cacao, soaked dates and all of the cream on top of the can of coconut milk. Gradually add up to 4 tbsp of the thinner coconut milk until your desired consistency is reached. This may take a few minutes to achieve a smooth yet thick mousse.
3. Spoon the mix into ramekin dishes, dividing into either two hefty or four slightly smaller portions. Leave to set in the fridge for at least 30 minutes.

Choosing the Perfect Nut Butter

We're busy women, so don't feel as if you have to make every single element of each recipe, from hand grinding your own nut butters to making your own chocolate from scratch. It's okay to delegate certain jobs to those who do it best. There are so many amazing brands out there who pride themselves on using quality, whole ingredients in their products. If you're shopping for peanut butter, make sure the only ingredient is peanuts! The same goes for your plant-based milks, dairy-free coconut yogurt and chocolate.

Why is there So Much Cacao in this Book?

Why? Because I'm a huge chocoholic. But seriously, raw cacao powder is the ultimate sanity restorer if you're avoiding tucking into that giant bar of chocolate hidden under your bed. It's antioxidant packed, extremely high in iron – a key nutrient for healthy ovulation – and gives you an instant mood boost, be it that time of the month or not.

You're Sweet Enough!

It's worth mentioning that your taste buds change over time, and as you add or remove things from your diet. Sweetness is subjective. What is super sweet and intensely chocolatey to me, someone who is hypersensitive to sugar in all its forms (sob), is tasteless to my chocolate-addict boyfriend. Experiment and have fun discovering new ways to naturally sweeten your foods, from adding a dash of maple syrup to your porridge, blending in sweet vegetables or simply adding a dusting of cinnamon.

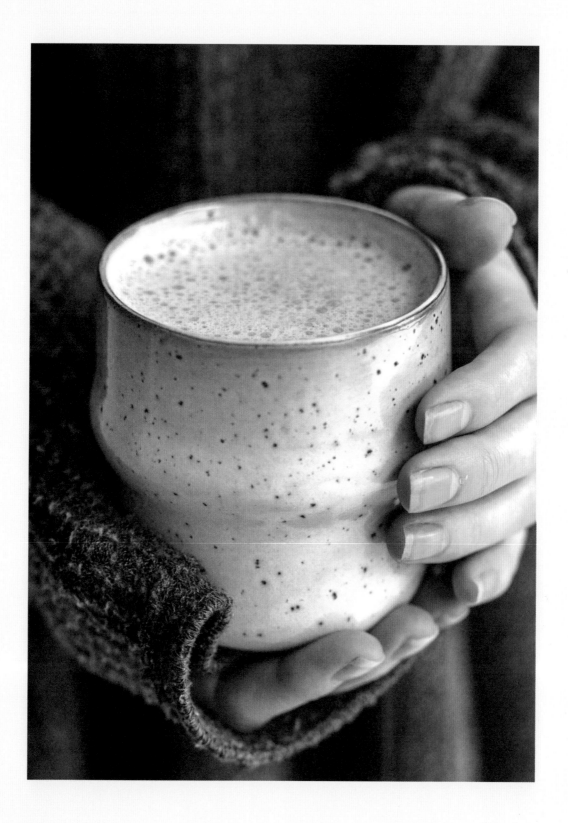

GRILLED NECTARINES WITH DAIRY-FREE COCONUT YOGURT, HAZELNUT BUTTER AND FLAKED ALMONDS

● ● ● ●

Dessert doesn't always have to be decadent layers of gateaux, cream-stuffed profiteroles or fancy crème brulée pots. Sometimes dessert is light, fresh and acts as the perfect full stop to a meal. Grilling up juicy nectarine halves is a fabulous way to look like you've made an effort, without really having to. Top with thick coconut yogurt, flaked almonds and a drizzle of hazelnut butter, and you have yourself a fool-proof barbecue pud, or an easy shared brunch side.

Serves 2

Prep: 2 minutes

Cook: 5 minutes

3 nectarines

2 tsp coconut oil

a few dollops of dairy-free coconut yogurt

2 tbsp Hazelnut Butter (see page 180)

a fistful of flaked almonds

1. Split each nectarine down the centre and remove the stone.
2. Heat a griddle pan and add the coconut oil. Place each nectarine half face down onto the griddle and cook for 5 minutes. Don't be tempted to touch them until the time is up.
3. Dress the grilled nectarines with a dollop of coconut yogurt, a drizzle of hazelnut butter and a sprinkling of flaked almonds, to serve.

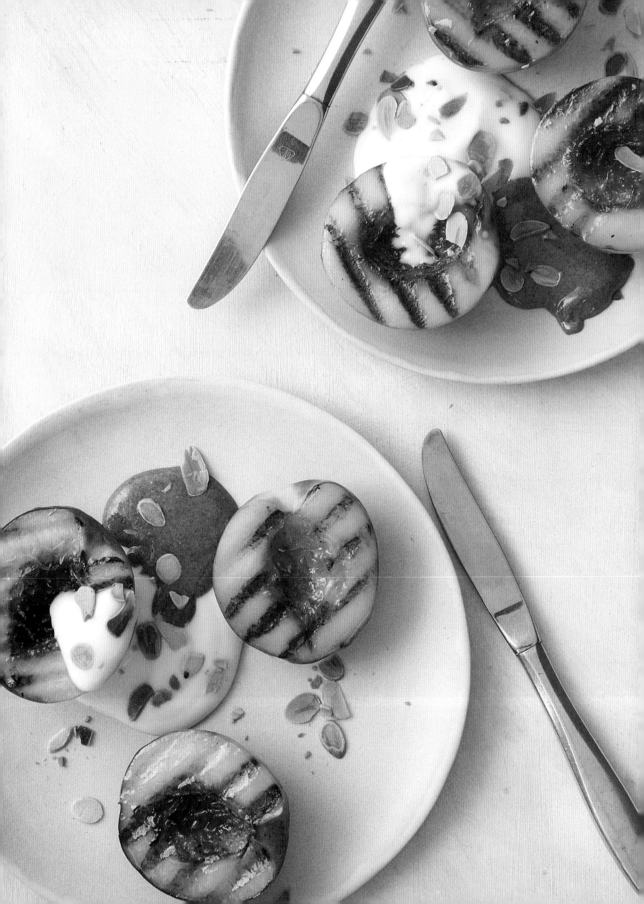

WATERMELON, STRAWBERRY AND FRESH MINT SALAD

● ● ● ●

Watermelon will always be a holiday fruit to me. Best enjoyed in warm climates, eaten fresh out of the hard shell, moments after being picked up from the local market. Better yet, chop up the watermelon and allow your surfaces to get super sticky as the juice pours out. Pair with lime, fresh mint and strawberries and you have the ultimate fuss-free summertime dessert.

Serves 4

Prep: 5 minutes

1 medium-sized watermelon

400 g (14 oz) strawberries, stalks removed and cut in half

1 small lime

6–8 fresh mint leaves

1 tbsp extra virgin olive oil

1. Peel the watermelon and chop into large slices and lay on a large platter. Top with the strawberries and grate over the zest from the lime. Chop the lime into quarters and leave on the side of the platter.

2. Make an easy mint drizzle by grounding up the fresh mint with the olive oil in a pestle and mortar, then drizzling over the top of the fruit.

Pick the perfect watermelon by holding it lovingly in your arms and gently tapping the side like a drum, a good watermelon should sound hollow.

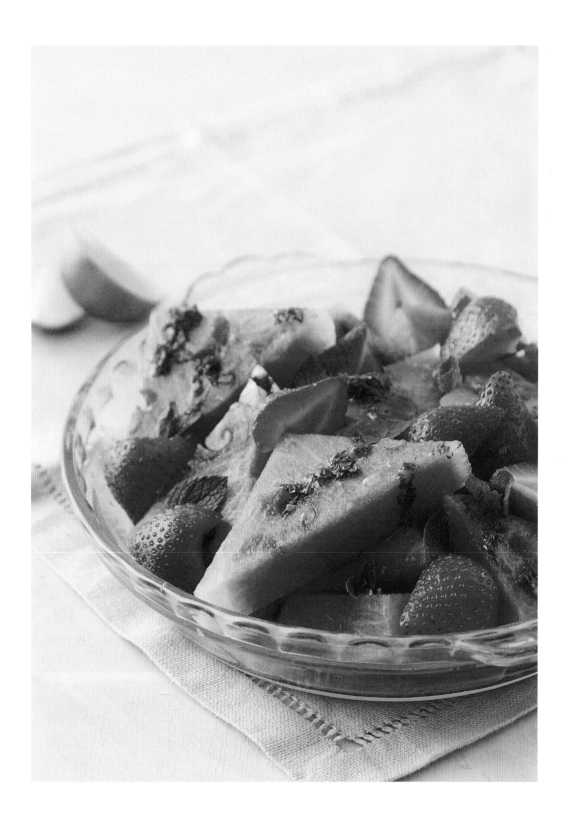

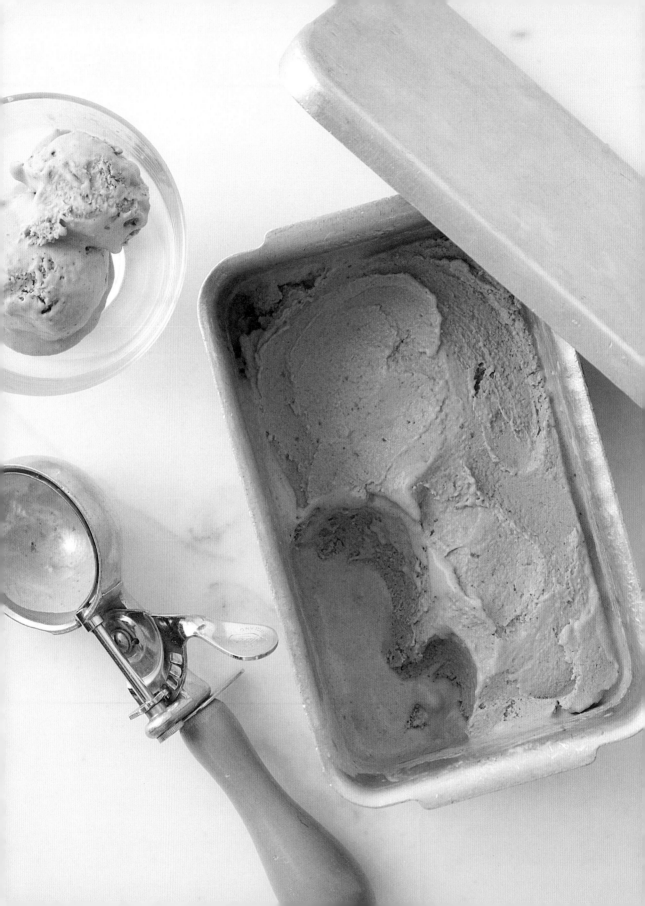

PISTACHIO ICE CREAM WITH OLIVE OIL

● ● ● ●

Pistachio is one of the most underrated flavours of ice cream, so it felt only right to squeeze in an easy, healthy recipe to give it some love. I like to substitute double cream for creamy, plant-based sources of fat including coconut milk, coconut oil and the nuts themselves, of course. Using medjool dates as the only form of sweetness ensures that instead of peaking into a post-sugar filled ice-cream-inflicted coma, you'll be glowing and satisfied without feeling stuffed.

Best enjoyed on a hot summer's day, finish with a sprinkling of roasted and crushed pistachios and extra virgin olive oil drizzled on top.

Makes: a small tub

Prep: 25 minutes, plus 30 minutes soaking and 3 hours freezing

Cook: 10 minutes

75 g (2 3/4 oz) pistachios

400 ml (14 oz) can full-fat coconut milk

2 tbsp coconut oil

2 medjool dates, stoned (soaked for at least 30 minutes in warm water)

½ tsp spirulina or matcha green tea powder

a light drizzle of extra virgin olive oil

1. Preheat the oven to 180°C/350°F/gas mark 4. Roast the pistachios on a baking tray for 10 minutes, then leave to completely cool.
2. Once cool, place the pistachios in a food processor or blender and blend until the oil breaks down and a butter forms. This can take up to 10 minutes and the mix should be runny.
3. Add the remaining ingredients, with the exception of the olive oil, as the blender runs for a good few minutes. You should have a silky-smooth mix by the end. Pour into a tub and place in the freezer to set.
4. Give the ice cream a good mix every hour or so until you no longer can. The ice cream should be solid after a three hour freeze, and will keep nicely for up to two weeks. Remove from the freezer for 10 minutes or so to defrost before eating. Drizzle with extra virgin olive oil, to serve.

While spirulina isn't essential in making this recipe, it does help deepen that gorgeous green colour slightly. It's also a good source of plant-based protein and rich in iron, making it a great addition to any hormone-healthy diet.

BLUEBERRY AND ALMOND LOAF WITH
LEMON CASHEW CREAM ICING

● ● ● ●

My search for low-sugar treats is never-ending. It often seems that every 'healthy' item sat on the supermarket shelves is packed full of hidden sugars. It's lead me to be stubborn with this recipe. I didn't want it packed full of sweetness, but it still had to be absolutely delicious. There is nothing worse than when your stomach starts to rumble mid-afternoon and the only thing you have to reach for is a something that'll leave you hungry within half-an-hour, so this blueberry and almond loaf is high in healthy fat to keep you satiated until dinner.

Makes one loaf

Prep: 15 minutes, plus overnight soaking

Cook: 30 minutes

2 ripe bananas

6 tbsp coconut oil

400 g (14 oz) ground almonds

30 g (1 oz) coconut flour

a scraping of seeds from a vanilla pod

1 tsp ground cinnamon (preferably Ceylon)

180 g (6 oz) blueberries, frozen or fresh

ICING

1 lemon

70 g (2¾ oz) cashews (soaked overnight in cold water)

5 tbsp almond milk (or your go-to plant-based milk)

1 tsp maple syrup (or your go-to liquid sweetener)

a fistful of toasted coconut flakes, to finish

1. Preheat the oven to 180°C/350°F/gas mark 4.
2. Mash the bananas in a large bowl. Melt the coconut oil in a bowl set over a pan of simmering water. Add the coconut oil to the bananas and mix.
3. Add the ground almonds, coconut flour, vanilla seeds and cinnamon and give everything a good mix. Lastly, add the frozen or fresh blueberries, folding in gently.
4. Tip the mix into a loaf tin that has been lined with baking parchment, smoothing down with the back of a spoon and making sure it's level and even. Place in the oven for 30 minutes to bake until golden brown on the top.
5. For the icing, grate the zest from the lemon and set aside. Squeeze the juice from the lemon. Combine the cashews, almond milk, 2 tsp lemon juice and syrup in a food processor or blender and blend for a good 5 minutes or so until completely smooth. Set aside. Ice the cake once cool and sprinkle over the lemon zest and toasted coconut flakes, to top.

The day before making, place your cashews in a bowl of water to soak overnight, to ensure a smooth, lump free icing.

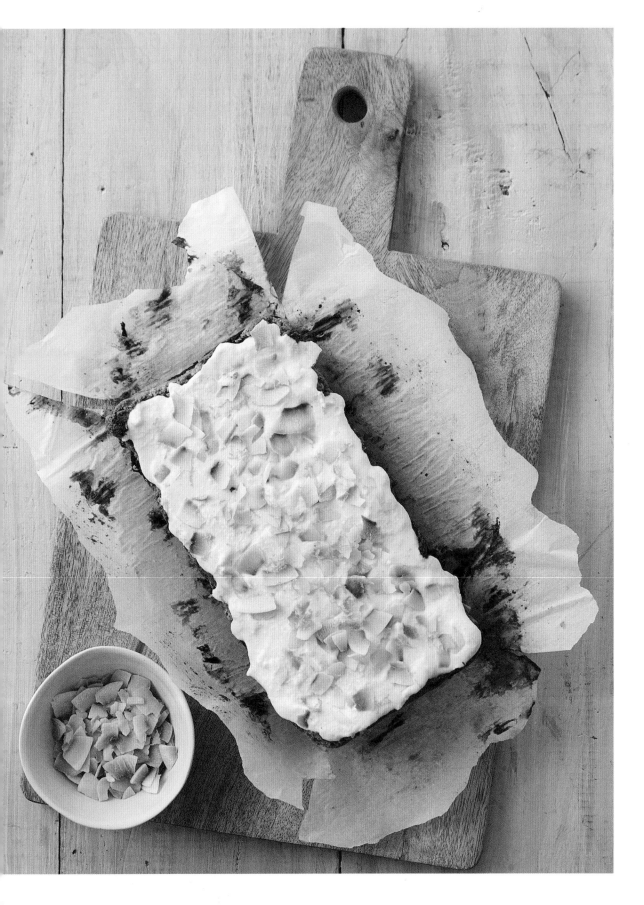

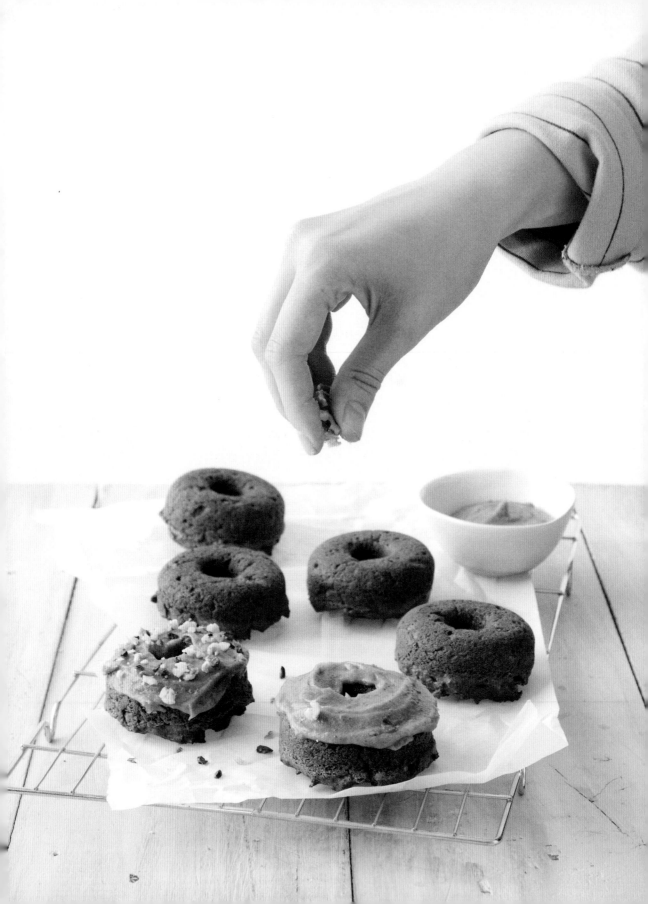

BANANA CINNAMON DOUGHNUTS WITH
SALTED COCONUT CARAMEL GLAZE

● ● ● ●

Scoffing sugar-coated, deep-fried cinnamon doughnuts by the seaside is one of the greatest pleasures in the world, and ending up with sticky fingers and sugar all down your front is absolutely worth it. Although life would be fabulous if this was an everyday occurrence, it probably wouldn't do wonders for your health. So, here you have it, a baked doughnut and banana bread hybrid, iced with creamy coconut caramel for a delicious healthier alternative. These doughnuts are crunchy on the outside, perfectly fluffy on the inside and taste just as good warm from the oven as they do after being glammed up with toppings.

Makes 6 doughnuts

Prep: 10 minutes

Cook: 25 minutes

2 tbsp milled flaxseed

1 large ripe banana (or 1½ small)

50 g (¼ cup) coconut oil, melted, plus extra for greasing

2 tbsp maple syrup

2 tbsp smooth almond butter

60 g (2 oz) ground almonds

100 g (3½ oz) buckwheat flour

½ tsp baking powder

½ tsp bicarbonate of soda

1½ tsp ground cinnamon (preferably Ceylon)

a pinch of salt

40 g (¼ cup) chopped walnuts

banana chips, crushed walnuts and cacao nibs, to top

SALTED COCONUT CARAMEL GLAZE

4 medjool dates, stoned (soaked in warm water for 30 minutes)

2 tbsp coconut cream (take from the top of a can of full-fat coconut milk)

1 tbsp coconut milk

a pinch of sea salt

1. Preheat the oven to 180°C/350°F/gas mark 4. Place the milled flaxseed in a small bowl along with 3 tablespoons water. Mash the banana in a large mixing bowl and add the melted coconut oil, maple syrup and almond butter, giving everything a good mix.

2. In a separate bowl, combine the all the dry ingredients, except the walnuts. Add to the bowl with the banana mix, thoroughly mix before adding the gooey flaxseed and the walnuts.

3. Give a doughnut tin a good greasing with a touch of coconut oil and evenly distribute the mix into each mould. Bake for 25 minutes then transfer to a wire rack to cool.

4. While the doughnuts are cooling, make the glaze. Place the soaked dates into a food processor or blender along with the coconut cream and a splash of the coconut milk. Blend for at least 5 minutes until the caramel is completely smooth and creamy. Add a pinch of sea salt at the very end. Ice the cooled doughnuts and decorate with a couple of banana chips, cacao nibs and crushed walnuts.

Don't panic if you don't have a doughnut tin, you can still make this recipe by spooning the mix into a lined muffin or cupcake tray instead.

COURGETTE AND CARROT SAVOURY MUFFINS ● ● ● ●

Baking doesn't always have to mean cupcakes and Victoria sponge; it can also mean hearty savoury snacks, packed full of flavour and spice. These fibre-filled wholesome muffins are exactly that, and fantastic if you're conscious about your sugar intake. Chickpea flour and coconut cream mean they are anything but dry, and grating in courgette and carrot is a fabulous way to get in extra veg. Serve warm, pulled apart with a thick layer of homemade pesto, or simply chuck one in your bag as you leave the house in the morning. They taste just as good cold.

Makes 6–8 muffins

Prep: 15 minutes

Cook: 35 minutes

2 tbsp milled flaxseed

1 large carrot

1 large courgette

1 garlic clove, minced

2 tbsp coconut
cream (take from
the top of a can)

5 tbsp extra virgin olive oil

50 g (roughly ½ cup)
of chickpea flour
(shop-bought or
homemade, see below)

70 g (¾ cup)
buckwheat flour

½ tsp baking powder

½ tsp bicarbonate of soda

½ tsp ground turmeric

½ tsp ground cumin

a fistful of thyme

a fistful of rosemary,
finely chopped

40 g (1½ oz) pumpkin and
sunflower seeds, to top

1. Preheat the oven to 180°C/350°F/gas mark 4.
2. Place the milled flaxseed in a small bowl with 4 tablespoons water and set aside.
3. Grate the carrot and courgette and blot away the excess moisture using a paper towel. Place the grated veg in a large bowl with the garlic, then add the coconut cream and olive oil.
4. In a separate bowl, combine all the dry ingredients, including the spices and herbs. Add this to the bowl with the grated veggies and mix thoroughly. Lastly, fold in the gooey flaxseed.
5. Line a muffin tin with paper cases and spoon in large dollops of the mixture. Sprinkle the seeds over the muffins and bake for 35 minutes, then leave to cool until warm.

To make your own chickpea flour, place 100 g/1 cup
dry chickpeas in a food processor or blender and
blitz for a good few minutes until a powder starts to
form, this may take a while. Pass through a fine sieve
and set aside until needed.

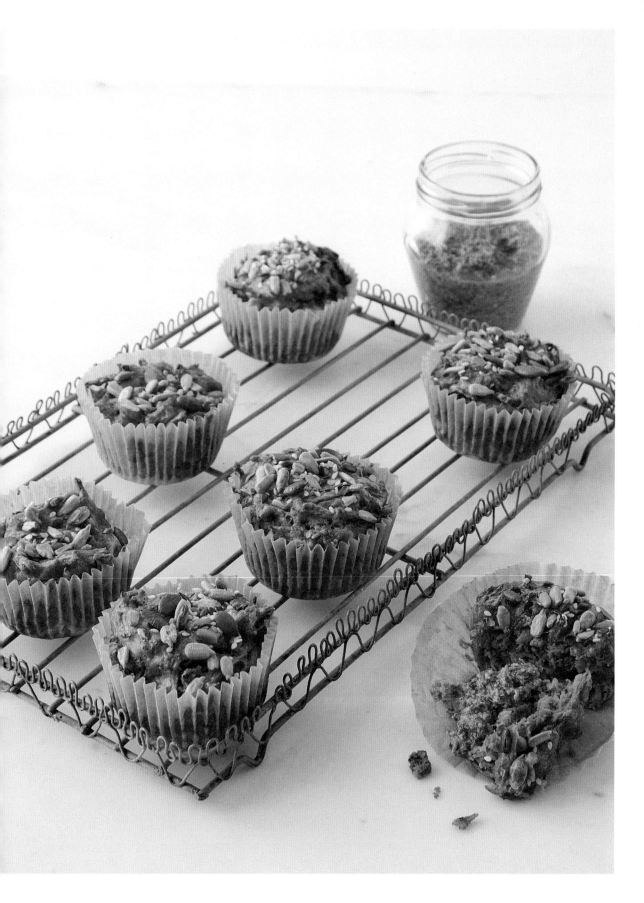

Basics

HOMEMADE PLANT-BASED MILKS

The ingredients list on the back of most plant-based milk cartons are a bit of a minefield. I am forever baffled as to why they add half the things they do, to what should be a basic staple. Making your own plant-based milk is not only cost effective; it's also undoubtedly better for you. It brings about a sense of pride that comes only from actually using that piece of muslin you've had hidden away for years. The soaking is the somewhat lengthy part of the overall process, often taking place overnight, however the rest is smooth sailing, as you simply blend and squeeze. From time to time, I'll take it a step further and get creative with flavourings, such as drool-worthy Chocolate Hazelnut Milk (see page 146) or a Iced Vanilla Cashew Chai (see page 140). For now, here are three basic plant-based milk recipes to get you started.

HAZELNUT MILK

● ● ● ●

**Makes: 500 ml
(2 cups)**

Prep: 10 minutes, plus overnight soaking

200 g (roughly 1½ cups) raw hazelnuts, soaked overnight

500 ml (2 cups) filtered water

a pinch of salt

CASHEW MILK

● ● ● ●

**Makes: 500 ml
(2 cups)**

Prep: 10 minutes, plus overnight soaking

200 g (roughly 1½ cups) raw cashews, soaked overnight

500 ml (2 cups) filtered water

a pinch of salt

HEMP MILK

● ● ● ●

**Makes: 500 ml
(2 cups)**

Prep: 10 minutes, plus overnight soaking

250 g (roughly 1½ cup) hulled hemp seeds, soaked overnight

500 ml (2 cups) filtered water

a pinch of salt

For all milks:

1. Ensure that you have soaked your chosen nut or seed overnight in water. When it comes to making the milk, thoroughly rinse your nuts or seeds and place into a food processor or blender with the filtered water. Blitz for a good few minutes.
2. Line a large jug with a muslin and fix it in place with a rubber band, making sure you can pour liquid into it and it will get caught in the cloth. Pour in the blitzed mixture, allowing all the liquid to drain through before lifting the cloth and squeezing out any excess. Store the milk in the fridge for up to three to four days.

Zero waste warrior? Save the nutty pulp
and bake it into brownies or add spoonfuls to
your morning smoothie.

NO NONSENSE PLANT-BASED BUTTERS

We often shy away from making our own staples, such as nut butters, as who really has the time? However, I was shocked at just how quick and easy it is to make basic ingredients like these. What's more, you have a greater control over what is going into each jar, ensuring that the only ingredient in your nut butter is, well, nuts. All you need is a food processor and a lidded jar to store the finished product.

Once you've got the basics down, the fun really begins. From adding raw cacao powder to hazelnut butter, to ground turmeric to your cashew blend, taking your nut butters to the next level is the ultimate way to liven up that fresh sourdough slice. Nut allergy? Fear not, sunflower and pumpkin seeds make amazing alternatives. Each keeps for at least a week in the fridge.

NUT BUTTER

Makes 1 small jar

Prep: 15 minutes

Cook: 5–10 minutes

200 g (7 oz) nuts (hazelnuts, almonds, cashews)

a pinch of sea salt

1. Preheat the oven to 180°C/350°F/gas mark 4
2. Spread the nuts out on a baking tray and bake for about 5–10 minutes, until the room starts to smell delightful.
3. Place the roasted nuts in a food processor or blender and blend. This will most likely take up to 10 minutes or so, and you should constantly be scraping the sides to ensure an even blend. You'll know it's ready once all the oils have been released and it starts to go runny.

SEED BUTTER

Makes 1 small jar

Prep: 20 minutes

Cook: 3–5 minutes

150 g (5½ oz) seeds (sunflower, pumpkin)

a pinch of sea salt

1. Gently toast your seeds of choice in a pan over a low heat until they start to pop and brown ever so slightly.
2. Place the toasted seeds in a food processor or blender and blend. This will most likely take up to 15 minutes or so, and you should constantly be scraping the sides to ensure an even blend. You'll know it's ready once all the oils have been released and it starts to go runny. Seed butters do take longer to reach the desired consistency than nuts do, so be patient.

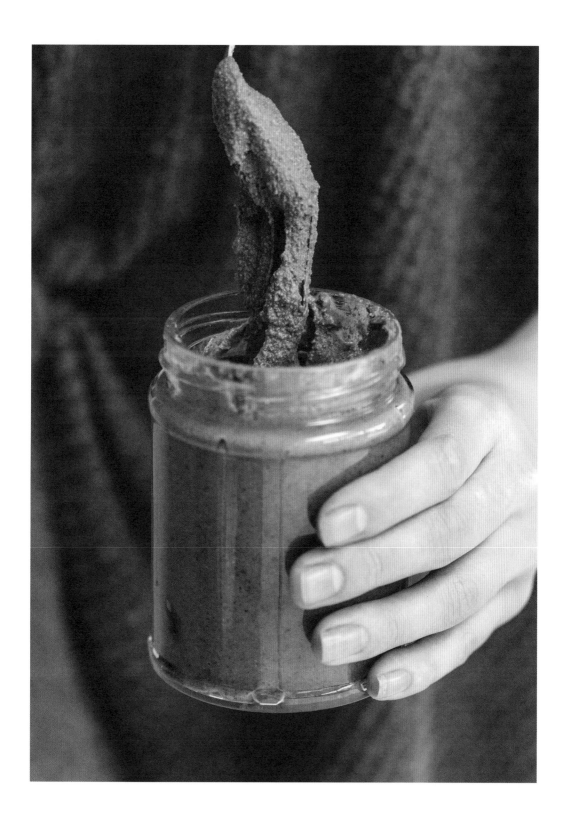

BASIL BRAZIL NUT PESTO

Brazil nuts are a truly marvellous nut. They're big, chunky and full of flavour. From a nutritional standpoint, they really stand their ground too. Brazil nuts are rich in selenium, a key nutrient in fighting inflammation, plus unsaturated fat and essential minerals, including magnesium, for promoting a healthy hormonal balance.

Makes 1 small jar

Prep: 5 minutes

70 g (½ cup) brazil nuts

a generous handful of basil

80 ml (⅓ cup) extra virgin olive oil

1 garlic clove, smashed

2 tbsp nutritional yeast (optional)

a light squeeze of lemon juice

salt and black pepper

1. Place all the ingredients in a food processor or blender and blitz until everything is combined and the brazil nuts are completely broken up. Feel free to add a touch more oil if you like a runnier pesto. Keeps for up to five days in a sealed container in the fridge.

CORIANDER NUT-FREE PESTO

Using fresh and fragrant coriander as a base for your pesto completely changes the game. It works fabulously over grilled summer veggies or stirred into hearty grains. Swapping nuts for toasted seeds means it is completely allergen-free, without compromising on that delicious chunky texture or missing out on the healthy plant-based fats.

Makes 1 small jar

Prep: 3–5 minutes

40 g (½ oz) pumpkin seeds

40 g (1½ oz) sunflower seeds

80 ml (⅓ cup) extra virgin olive oil

a generous fistful of fresh coriander

1 garlic clove

2 tbsp nutritional yeast

salt and black pepper

1. Toast the seeds gently in a pan until they begin to pop. Add the seeds and remaining ingredients to a food processor or blender and blitz until everything is combined and the seeds have been broken up. Keeps for up to five days in a sealed container in the fridge.

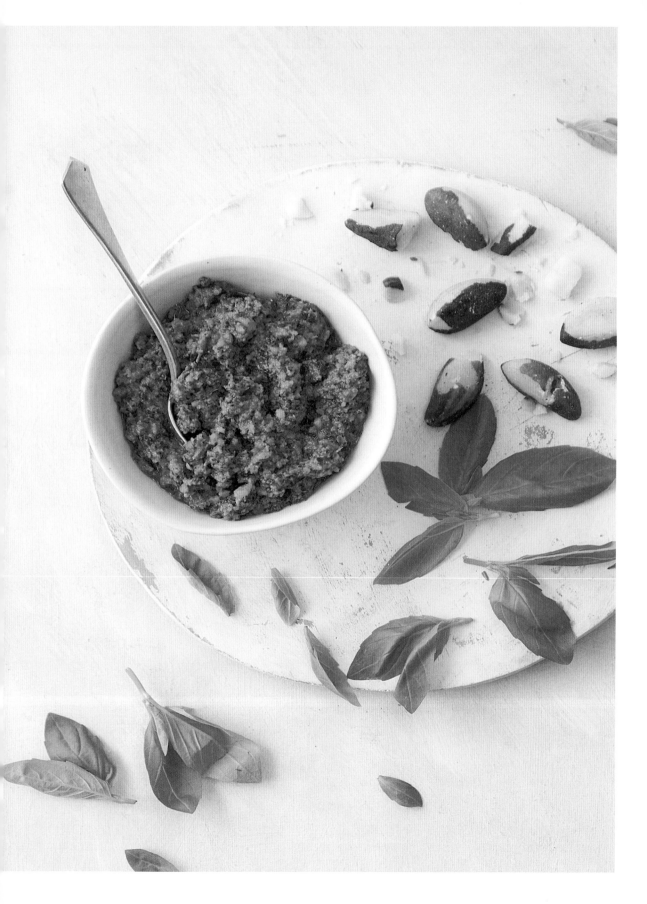

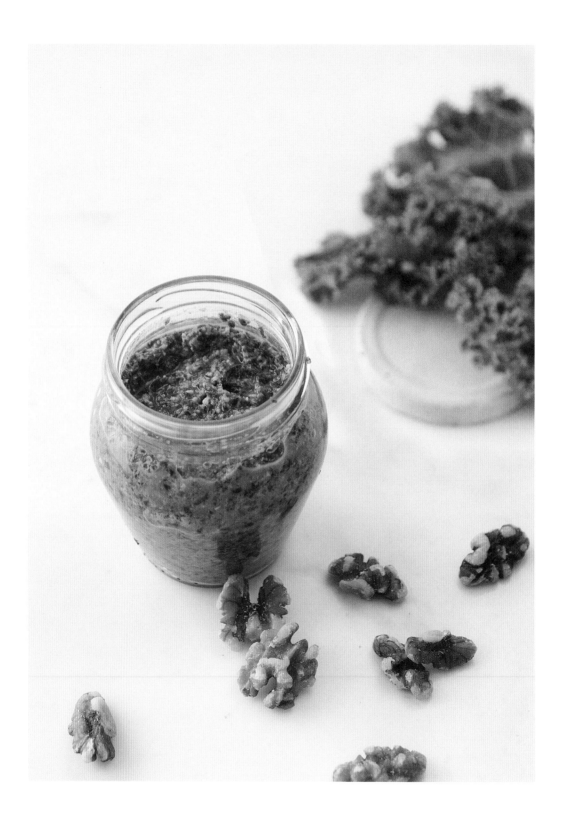

KALE AND GARLIC PESTO

● ● ● ●

Kale is one of the most nutrient-dense foods around, but sometimes we just can't face another boring kale salad. Instead, blitz it into a rich, garlicky pesto, perfect for livening up any bowl of spaghetti. I like to throw in a handful of walnuts, as they are rich in essential Omega-3s, essential for both brain and heart health, as well as aiding in healthy digestion.

Makes 1 small jar

Prep: 5 minutes

a large handful
of fresh kale

1 garlic clove, peeled

50 g (1¾ oz) raw walnuts

80 ml (⅓ cup) extra virgin
olive oil or avocado oil

2 tbsp nutritional yeast

1. Place all the ingredients into a food processor or blender and blitz until everything is combined and the kale and walnuts are completely broken up. Feel free to add a touch more oil if you like a runnier pesto. Keeps for up to five days in a sealed container in the fridge.

GREEN CORIANDER CREAM DRESSING

● ● ● ●

If there was ever a salad dressing to make you visibly radiate health, it's this one. This green coriander cream is chock-a-block with glorious ingredients guaranteed to make you glow. It's high fat and packed full of gorgeous greens, from spinach to fresh and fragrant coriander. I chuck in a few overflowing tablespoons of hemp seeds, as they're rich in GLA, an Omega-6 fatty acid known for its hormone balancing effects. They're also a great source of plant-based protein. Dollop on the side of sharing plates of roasted vegetables, fold into zesty quinoa salads or simply serve as a dip for crunchy vegetable sticks.

Makes a small bowl

Prep: 5 minutes

1 ripe avocado

a small fistful of
fresh coriander

3 tbsp extra virgin olive oil

a fistful of spinach leaves

2 tbsp hemp seeds

a squeeze of lemon juice

salt and black pepper

1. Slice the avocado down the centre and remove the stone. Scoop out the flesh into a food processor or blender and add the remaining ingredients. Blend until completely smooth and creamy, this may take a few minutes. Keeps for up to five days in a sealed container in the fridge.

TURMERIC AND COCONUT DRESSING

● ● ● ●

If you're a fan of garlic butter, I have no doubt you'll absolutely adore this turmeric and coconut dressing. Not only is it ridiculously moreish, it's also highly anti-inflammatory, from the golden turmeric and the extra virgin olive oil, as well as being antibacterial and antiviral from the garlic. A generous drizzle of this dressing tossed through your salads and grains will keep illness at bay, hormones in harmony and transform any meal. One taste of this lovely high-fat gloriousness and you'll never want to buy salad dressing again.

Makes a small bowl

Prep: 5 minutes

4 tbsp full-fat coconut milk (from can)

½ tbsp ground turmeric powder

1 garlic clove, minced

2 tbsp nutritional yeast

1 tbsp extra virgin olive oil

salt and black pepper

1. Place all the ingredients into a food processor or blender and blitz until completely smooth and creamy. Pour over salads or into a small pot ready to dip veggies into. Keeps for up to five days in a sealed container in the fridge.

HOMEMADE HUMMUS

Hummus is one of those dips that can be used in a magnitude of different ways, from spreading thickly in chunky roasted vegetable wraps, as a dip for tortilla chips (see page 130) or simply dolloped on the side of a wholesome wholegrain salad. Hummus makes everything better. Making it yourself is also surprisingly easy, and much more cost effective than the shop-bought stuff. Once you've got the base down, you can really go to town on flavours. From your basic creamy cumin spiced dip, sweet beetroot to maple roast carrot, it's a truly fabulous way to cram in those vibrant veggies and use up any leftover produce sitting in your fridge.

QUICK AND SIMPLE HUMMUS

Makes 1 small bowl

Prep: 10 minutes

400 g (14 oz) can chickpeas

1 tbsp tahini

½ tsp ground cumin

120 ml (½ cup) extra virgin olive oil

1 garlic clove

a squeeze of lemon juice

salt and black pepper

1. Start by draining and thoroughly rinsing the chickpeas. Next remove the skins by gently pinching the edges and letting the chickpeas pop out. This will give an extra smooth hummus.
2. Place the skinned chickpeas in a food processor or blender along with the remaining ingredients and blitz until smooth. This may take a couple of minutes or so, depending on desired consistency. Keeps for up to five days in a sealed container in the fridge.

From top to bottom: Quick and Simple Hummus; Maple Roasted Carrot Hummus.

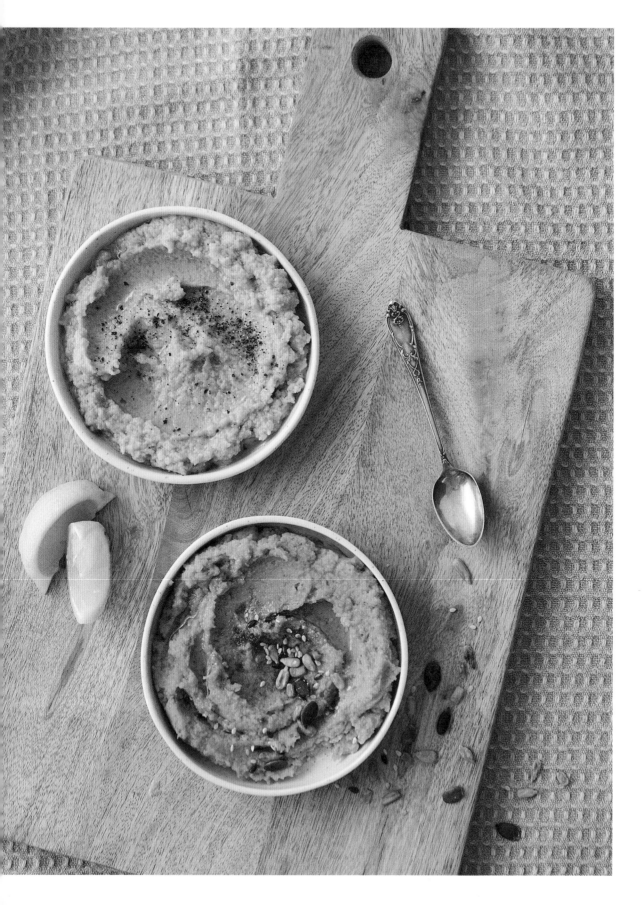

MAPLE ROASTED CARROT HUMMUS

● ● ● ●

Makes 1 small bowl

Prep: 15 minutes

Cook: 25 minutes

2 small carrots (total
weight about 200 g/
7 oz), roughly chopped

a drizzle of avocado oil

1 tsp maple syrup

400 g (14 oz) can
chickpeas

1 tbsp tahini

½ tsp ground cumin

120 ml (½ cup) extra
virgin olive oil

1 garlic clove

a squeeze of lemon juice

salt and black pepper

1. Preheat the oven to 180°C/350°F/gas mark 4.
2. Place the carrots on a roasting tray with a drizzle of avocado oil and
   the maple syrup, ensuring each piece is coated. Roast for about
   25 minutes until soft and golden.
3. Drain and rinse the chickpeas. Next remove the skins by gently
   pinching the edges and letting the chickpeas pop out. This will give
   an extra smooth hummus.
4. Place the skinned chickpeas in a food processor or blender along
   with the remaining ingredients, including the roasted carrots.
   Blitz until smooth. Keeps for up to five days in a sealed container
   in the fridge.

For the smoothest, creamiest consistency,
peel your chickpeas before adding into the food
processor. It doesn't take long, and is done simply by
pinching the chickpeas in between your fingers.

From left to right: Sweet
Beet Hummus; Kale and
Garlic Pesto; Maple Roasted
Carrot Hummus.

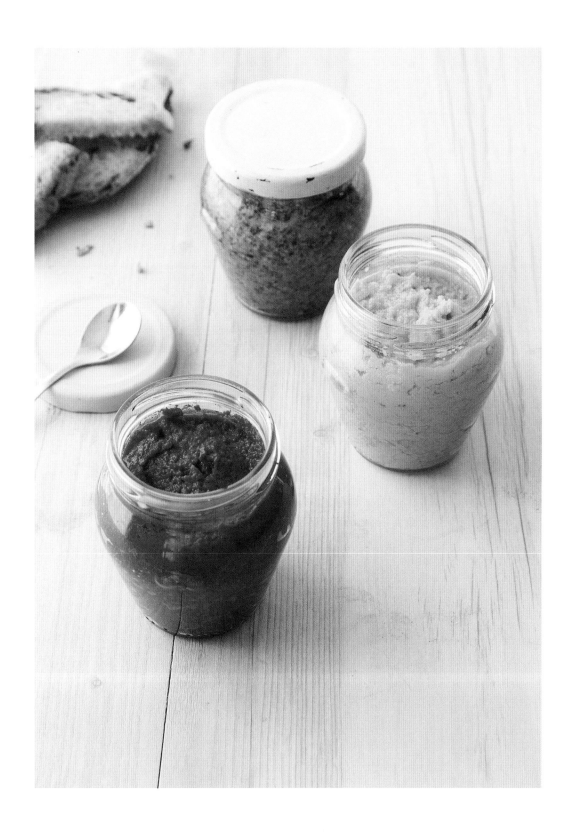

CHAPTER 4

And Finally

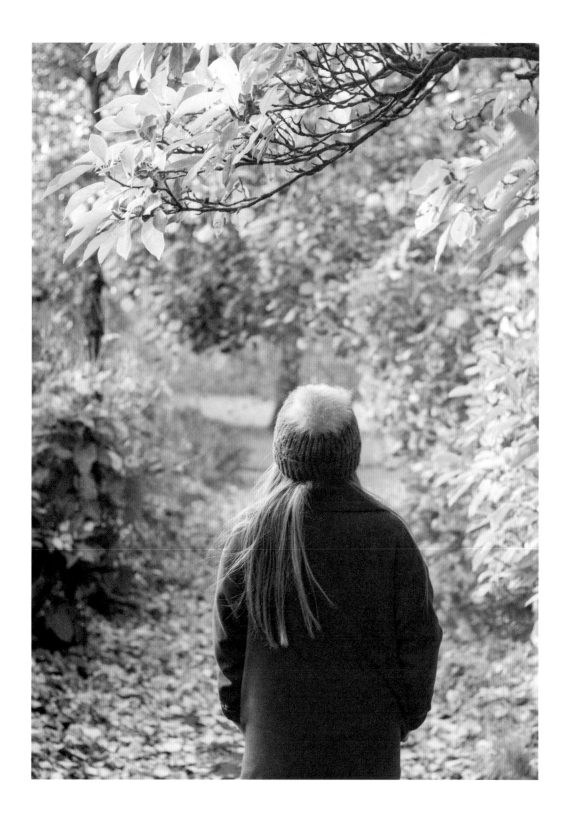

MEAL GUIDES

I've pulled together a week's worth of meals to show you the basics of what a hormone-healthy diet looks like. Each day is packed full of foods that will make you feel amazing, with tips on where you can make double portions of your dinner the night before, so you'll always have food for the next day. Follow them loosely, or religiously, it's completely up to you.

Sunday
Brunch: Veggie Breakfast Tray Bake (see page 89)
Snack: Sunshine Juice (see page 65)
Dinner: Lentil Shepherd's Pie with Creamy Cashew and Sweet Potato Mash (see page 120) – make a big portion for lunch tomorrow
Still peckish: Lemon and Black Sesame Seed Nourish Ball (see page 149)
Prep: Prepare the sweet potato and freeze overnight for Monday's breakfast (see page 62). Soak cashews and store in the fridge for Thursday's lunch (see page 99). Make three portions of quinoa.

Move: Relax! It's Sunday

Monday
Breakfast: Chocolate Almond Butter Smoothie (see page 62)
Lunch: Lentil Shepherd's Pie with Creamy Cashew and Sweet Potato Mash (leftover)
Snack: Lemon and Black Sesame Seed Nourish Ball (leftover)
Dinner: Wild Mushroom Ragu with Creamy Courgetti (see page 107) – make a double portion of ragu
Still peckish: A bowl of berries with dairy-free coconut yogurt, cinnamon and almond butter

Move: Start the week with an early morning spin class. If you are in your luteal or menstrual phase, opt for slow flow yoga instead.

Tuesday
Breakfast: Blueberry Breakfast Smoothie (see page 63) – make a double portion

Lunch: Wild Mushroom Ragu (leftover) with creamy courgetti (make fresh)
Snack: Golden Coconut Milk (see page 138) and a bowl of berries
Dinner: Delicata Squash and Black Rice Salad (see page 96) – make a double portion
Still peckish: Lemon and Black Sesame Seed Nourish Ball (leftover)

Move: Go for a long evening walk with your best friend, or furry friend!

Wednesday

Breakfast: Sprouted Quinoa Porridge (see page 71) – quinoa prepped on Sunday
Lunch: Delicata Squash and Black Rice Salad (leftover)
Snack: Liver-Supporting Green Juice (see page 65)
Dinner: Chunky Veggie and Quinoa Soup (see page 102) – quinoa prepped on Sunday
Still peckish: Whip up a Sweet Potato Chocolate Mousse (see page 161) for dessert

Move: Hit your local swimming pool and get some lengths in before work

Thursday

Breakfast: Blueberry Breakfast Smoothie (leftover)
Lunch: Chilled Avocado and Pea Soup (see page 99) with white quinoa prepped on Sunday
Snack: Courgette and Carrot Savoury Muffin (see page 174)
Dinner: Roasted Carrot, Pearled Spelt and Orange Salad (see page 92) – make a double portion
Still peckish: Coconut Butter Cup (see page 150)
Prep: Overnight Teff Breakfast Bowl (see page 74) for Friday's breakfast

Move: Go for a quick jog or try out an online Pilates class

Friday

Breakfast: Overnight Teff Breakfast Bowl (prepped Thursday evening)
Lunch: Roasted Carrot, Pearled Spelt and Orange Salad (leftover)
Snack: Coconut Butter Cup (leftover)
Dinner: Brown Rice Spaghetti with Spring Greens (see page 108)
Still peckish: Courgette and Carrot Savoury Muffin (leftover)

Move: Take a yoga class and Om your way into the weekend

Saturday

Breakfast: Cherry Cacao Teff Pancakes (see page 86)
Lunch: Roasted Fennel, Rocket and Wild Rice Salad (see page 94)
Snack: A bowl of berries with dairy-free coconut yogurt, cinnamon and almond butter
Dinner: Beetroot and Carrot Burgers with Satay Slaw (see page 126) and a side of Zesty Chargrilled Broccoli (see page 135)
Still peckish: Mushroom Hot Chocolate with Coconut Cream (see page 139)

Move: Lift some weights or attend a fun dance class with a friend

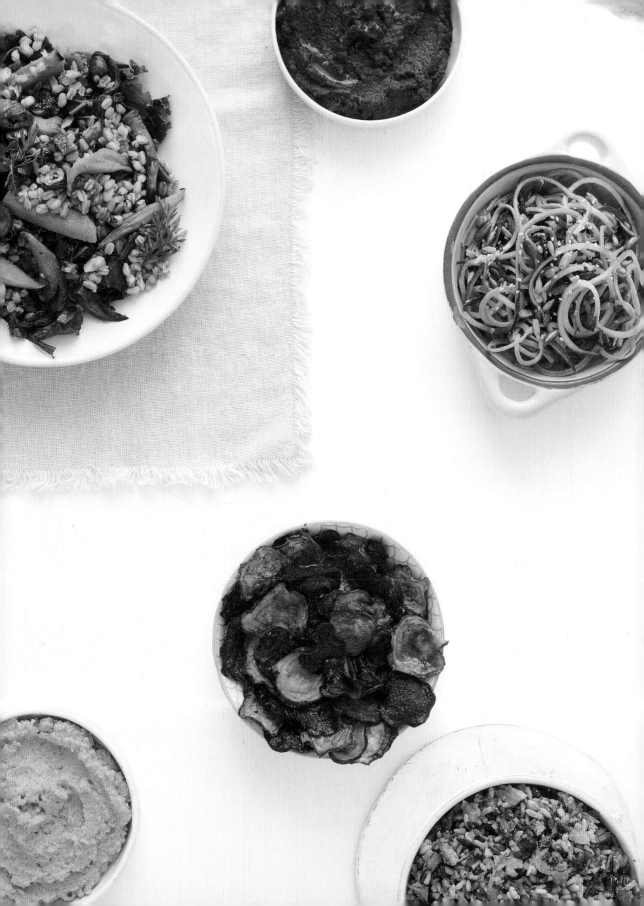

GLOSSARY OF HORMONAL CONDITIONS

Adenomyosis

A condition in which the uterine lining grows into the muscular wall of the uterus causing the uterine walls to thicken, and the uterus to enlarge. Similar to endometriosis, this condition causes extremely painful and heavy periods, and is difficult to diagnose because it can often overlap with endometriosis and uterine fibroids.

Amenorrhea

A condition where a woman is missing her period completely. Primary amenorrhea is when menstruation has not naturally started by the age of 16. Secondary amenorrhea occurs when a woman has not menstruated for 3–6 months when she previously had regular periods, or 9 months if she previously had irregular periods.

Endometriosis

When endometrial cells that usually grow inside the uterus are found outside of the uterus, often on organs in and around the pelvis like the fallopian tubes, the surface of the uterus and the lining of the pelvic cavity. This condition can cause extremely painful periods, heavy menstrual flow, long periods, bowel and urinary disorders and pain during sex.

Hyperthyroidism

This is when the thyroid is overactive or producing too much thyroid hormone (T4, T3 or both). It is a lot less common than Hypothyroidism. Hyperthyroidism is most commonly seen in those with Grave's disease, which is an auto-immune disorder that occurs when the body's immune system releases antibodies that stimulate the thyroid to produce more and more thyroid hormone.

Hypothyroidism

This is when the thyroid is underactive or producing too little thyroid hormone (T4, T3 or both). Hashimoto's Thyroiditis is an autoimmune condition in which the body produces antibodies that mistakenly attack healthy thyroid tissue, and it is the most prevalent cause of hypothyroidism.

Infertility

The inability to get pregnant naturally during normal reproduction years, due to lack of ovulation, physical problems with the reproductive organs or other conditions.

Polycystic Ovarian Syndrome (PCOS)

A condition that affects roughly 15–20 percent of women worldwide and approximately 1 in 5 women in the UK. It's also earned the honour of being the most common endocrine disorder in women of reproductive age. PCOS is a bit of a misnomer, because it's not a single condition, but rather, a collection of symptoms that include high levels of androgens or male hormones, polycystic ovaries, male pattern hair loss, hair growth on the face or other body parts, acne and irregular or absent periods.

Premenstrual Dysphoric Disorder (PMDD)

A more severe form of PMS, which includes symptoms severe enough to disrupt a woman's daily life. PMDD is often confused with clinical depression, but the difference is that PMDD-related mood changes always occur in conjunction with menstruation.

Premenstrual Syndrome (PMS)

Refers to the group of cyclical physical and emotional symptoms that occur during the latter half of the menstrual cycle. What underlies PMS is an imbalance between the two main female sex hormones oestrogen and progesterone, which fluctuate throughout a woman's cycle. These hormones also heavily influence brain chemicals including serotonin, dopamine and oxytocin, which all affect mood and even gut health.

Uterine fibroids

Non-cancerous growths found inside or outside of the uterus, that often show up during a woman's childbearing years. Fibroids can cause heavy or prolonged bleeding in some women, spotting between periods and severe period pain.

RECIPE INDEX

GENERAL INDEX

oestrogen *cont.*
  detoxing from the body 26,
    32, 52
  luteal phase 42
  melatonin and 35
  ovulatory phase 41
omega-3 fatty acids 52, 54, 55
ovaries 17, 22, 40
ovulation 27, 40, 54, 160
  ovulatory phase 41

pancreas 17, 18–19, 23
pasta 51
perfume 38
perimenopause 13, 22, 39
periods *see* menstruation
phytic acid 92
Pilates 36
pineal 17, 18
pituitary 17, 18
plant-based milks 160, 178
pollutants 26–7
Polycystic Ovarian Syndrome
  (PCOS) 9, 25, 26, 47, 52,
  66, 115, 199
prebiotics 32, 66
pregnenolone 19, 24
progesterone 19, 21, 27
  cortisol and insulin
    imbalance 23, 24
  luteal phase 42
  melatonin and 35
  menstrual phase 43
  perimenopause 22
  vitamin C and 47

protein 54
protein powders 48
puberty 20, 21
pumpkin seeds 47, 158

quinoa 47

ready meals 50
REM sleep 34
retinol 54

salmon 55
sanitary products 37
screen time 31, 35, 44
sea veg 48
seeds 47, 54, 92
  seed butters 180
selenium 21, 54, 182
serotonin 32, 42
sex hormones 18, 19, 21
shampoo 38
skin, toxins and 37
sleep 31, 34–5, 143
spelt 122
stress 31, 34
stress hormones 18, 23–4
styling products 38
sugar 33, 41, 50, 64
sulforaphane 94
sunscreen 37
superfoods 46–8, 115
supplements 52
sweet potatoes 47

sweetness 160
swimming 36

taste buds 160
tea, herbal 33, 47
teff 74
testosterone 18, 19, 21, 23, 24,
  27, 40, 42
thyroid 17, 18, 22, 23, 24–5
toothpaste 37
toxins 26–7, 37

vegetables
  cruciferous 30, 46, 135
  juices 64
  sea veg 48
vitamins
  A 21, 54
  B-complex 21, 33, 52, 64
  B12 21, 54, 55
  C 21, 47
  D 21
  E 21, 47, 155

walking 36
water 30, 32, 33
wholegrains 47, 85

yoga 36
yogurt, dairy-free coconut 46–7, 85

zinc 21, 54, 74, 92

RESOURCES

Brands I love

Coconut Milk Yogurt
CoYo
http://coyo.com
Key stockists: Waitrose, Ocado, Sainsbury's,
Wholefoods Market, Planet Organic

Chocolate
Ombar
https://www.ombar.co.uk/
Key stockists: Waitrose, Ocado, Wholefoods
Market, Planet Organic, As Nature Intended

Loving Earth
https://lovingearth.co/
Key stockists: Planet Organic, Holland &
Barrett

Pana Chocolate
https://panachocolate.com/
Key stockists: Planet Organic, As Nature
Intended

For Non-Dairy milk
Oatly
https://www.oatly.com/
Key stockists: Waitrose, Ocado, Sainsbury's,
Tesco, Asda, Morrisons

Plenish
https://www.plenishdrinks.com/
Key stockists: Waitrose, Ocado, Sainsbury's,
Asda, Planet Organic

Rude Health
https://rudehealth.com/
Key stockists: Waitrose, Ocado, Sainsbury's,
Tesco, Asda, Morrisons

For Nut Butter
Meridian
http://www.meridianfoods.co.uk/
Key stockists: Waitrose, Ocado, Sainsbury's,
Tesco, Asda, Morrisons

Pip and Nut
https://www.pipandnut.com/
Key stockists: Ocado, Sainsbury's, Tesco,
Asda, Morrisons, Holland & Barrett

Biona
http://www.biona.co.uk/
Key stockists: Ocado, Planet Organic, Holland
& Barrett, Amazon

For Protein Powder
Welleco
https://www.welleco.co.uk/
Ket stockists: Wholefoods Market, Space NK,
Net-A-Porter

Naturya
https://naturya.com/
Key stockists: Waitrose, Ocado, Sainsbury's,
Holland & Barratt, Planet Organic, Wholefood
Market, As Nature Intended

Garden of Life
https://www.gardenoflife.com/
Key stockists: Planet Organic, Amazon

For Superfoods
Naturya
https://naturya.com/
Key stockists: Waitrose, Ocado, Sainsbury's,
Holland & Barratt, Planet Organic, Wholefood
Market, As Nature Intended

ACKNOWLEDGEMENTS

Kiki Health
https://kiki-health.com/
Key stockists: Planet Organic, Amazon

For Medicinal Mushrooms
Hybrid Herbs
https://www.hybridherbs.co.uk/
Key stockists: Planet Organic, Revital

For Herbal Tea
Pukka
https://www.pukkaherbs.com/
Waitrose, Ocado, Sainsbury's, Tesco, Asda,
Morrisons

Yogi Tea
https://www.yogitea.com/
Key stockists: Waitrose, Ocado, Holland &
Barratt, Planet Organic

For Supplements
Viridian
https://www.viridian-nutrition.com/
Key stockists: Planet Organic, Neal's Yard
Remedies

Terranova
http://www.terranovahealth.com/
Key stockists: Planet Organic, Amazon

Where to Shop
Indigo Herbs
https://www.indigo-herbs.co.uk/
Planet Organic (You can shop online too if
you're outside of London)
https://www.planetorganic.com/

To my brilliant editor Philippa, for being an absolute dream to work with. Thank you for making sense of my rambles and making my wildest dream come true.

Simon and Veronica, for making recipes on paper turn into photographic masterpieces, and for cooking and styling each dish better than I ever could.

Nicole, thank you for your amazing words. Our philosophies around hormone health align so perfectly, and it's been great having you on board for this project.

My parents, for supporting me regardless of the state of the kitchen, hefty food shops and endless taste tests. I couldn't have achieved any of this without you and I am so grateful for everything you have done, and continue to do, for me.

Ben. You are truly wonderful and I couldn't imagine working towards my goals without you by my side.

Clive, thank you for your recipe testing and detailed feedback. Thank you for your continued faith in everything I do.

To all the women in my life who inspire me every single day. To Bea, Lucy, Lily, Chloe, Zoe and to all the Betties. Thank you for being the most supportive best friends a girl could wish for.

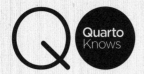

Brimming with creative inspiration, how-to projects and useful information to enrich your everyday life, Quarto Knows is a favourite destination for those pursuing their interests and passions. Visit our site and dig deeper with our books into your area of interest: Quarto Creates, Quarto Cooks, Quarto Homes, Quarto Lives, Quarto Drives, Quarto Explores, Quarto Gifts, or Quarto Kids.

First published in 2019 by White Lion Publishing,
an imprint of The Quarto Group.
The Old Brewery, 6 Blundell Street
London, N7 9BH,
United Kingdom
T (0)20 7700 6700

www.QuartoKnows.com

A catalogue record for this book is available from the British Library.
ISBN 978 1 78131 860 7
Ebook ISBN 978 1 78131 861 4

10 9 8 7 6 5 4 3 2 1

Design by Paileen Currie
Photography by Simon Pask
Food Styling by Veronica Eijo

Printed in China

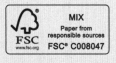

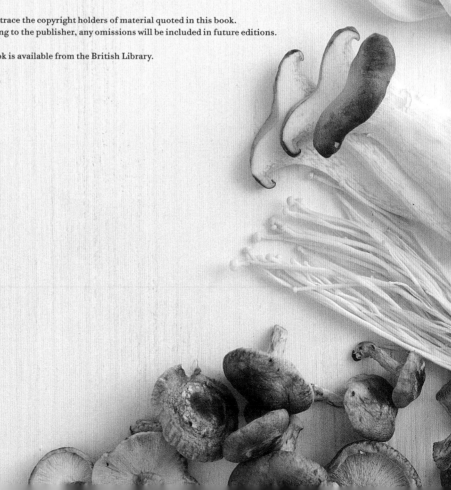

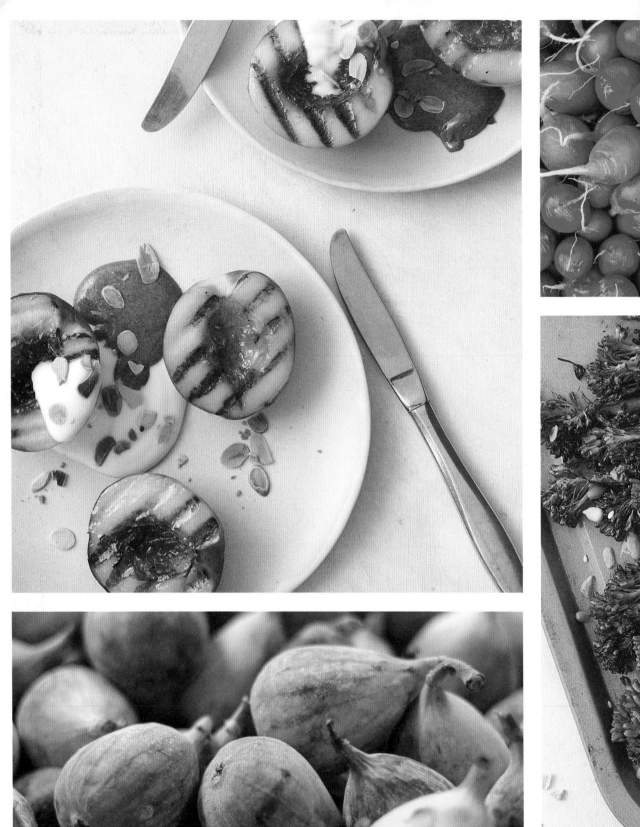